Mitigating the Effects of Blast-Related Burn Injuries from Prolonged Field Care to Rehabilitation and Resilience

Proceedings and Expert Findings from a U.S. Department of Defense International State-of-the-Science Meeting

EMILY HOCH, SAMANTHA MCBIRNEY, CHARLES C. ENGEL, TEPRING PIQUADO

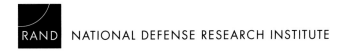

NATIONAL DEFENSE RESEARCH INSTITUTE

For more information on this publication, visit www.rand.org/t/CFA807-2

Library of Congress Cataloging-in-Publication Data is available for this publication.
ISBN: 978-1-9774-0618-7

Published by the RAND Corporation, Santa Monica, Calif.
© Copyright 2020 RAND Corporation
RAND® is a registered trademark.

Support RAND
Make a tax-deductible charitable contribution at
www.rand.org/giving/contribute

www.rand.org

Preface

This document represents the complete proceedings of the Ninth Department of Defense International State-of-the-Science Meeting (SoSM) on Blast Injury Research, held from March 3 to March 5, 2020, at the Arlington, Virginia, office of the RAND Corporation. The topic of the ninth SoSM was "Mitigating the Effects of Blast-Related Burn Injuries from Prolonged Field Care to Rehabilitation and Resilience." The SoSM aims to identify knowledge gaps in blast-injury research; ensure that the U.S. Department of Defense (DoD) medical research programs address existing gaps; foster collaboration; promote information-sharing on the latest research; and identify short-term, intermediate, and long-term actions to prevent, mitigate, and treat blast injuries. Participants and presenters consisted of scientists, clinicians, and policymakers from DoD, including the Departments of the Army, Navy, and Air Force; the Marine Corps; the National Institutes of Health; and the U.S. Department of Veterans Affairs; as well as representatives from academia and industry and scholars from several different countries. This research should be of interest to senior military and medical leaders.

The Human Subjects Protection Committee (HSPC) is RAND's institutional review board to review research involving human subjects, as required by federal regulations. RAND's Federalwide Assurance for the Protection of Human Subjects (FWA00003425, effective until June 22, 2023) serves as the organization's assurance of compliance with the regulations of 17 federal departments and agencies. According to this assurance, the HSPC is responsible for review of all research, regardless of the source of funding. The views of sources used in this study are solely their own and do not represent the official policy or position of DoD or the U.S. government.

This research was sponsored by the U.S. Army Medical Research and Development Command and the DoD Blast Injury Research Coordinating Office and conducted within the Forces and Resources Policy Center of the RAND National Security Research Division (NSRD), which operates the National Defense Research Institute (NDRI), a federally funded research and development center sponsored by the Office of the Secretary of Defense, the Joint Staff, the Unified Combatant Commands, the Navy, the Marine Corps, the defense agencies, and the defense intelligence enterprise.

For more information on the RAND Forces and Resources Policy Center, see www.rand.org/nsrd/frp or contact the director (contact information is provided on the webpage).

Contents

Figures and Tables

Figures

Tables

Acknowledgments

The members of the RAND research team gratefully acknowledge Dr. Mark Dertzbaugh and Dr. Raj Gupta at the Blast Injury Research Coordinating Office for their comments, guidance, and support for this project. They also extend their thanks to the members of the State-of-the-Science Meeting (SoSM) planning committee (see Appendix E). These individuals helped the research team identify expert panel candidates, advised on invited speaker topics, nominated speakers, reviewed meeting abstract submissions, provided input on the working group discussion questions, helped refine the SoSM agenda, and moderated the SoSM question-and-answer panels.

The RAND research team derived tremendous inspiration and support from the expert panel. Each expert panelist chaired a working group, and key parts of this document (findings, conclusions, and recommendations) were written in close consultation with these respected scholars:

- Leopoldo (Lee) C. Cancio, M.D., F.A.C.S., FCCM, Director, U.S. Army Burn Center at the U.S. Army Institute of Surgical Research, San Antonio, Texas
- William Scott Dewey, PT, CHT, Chief of Rehabilitation, U.S. Army Burn Center, San Antonio, Texas
- Matthias Donelan, M.D., Chief of Staff, Shriners Hospitals for Children, Boston, Massachusetts
- Nicole S. Gibran, M.D., F.A.C.S., Associate Dean for Research and Graduate Education, University of Washington School of Medicine, Seattle, Washington
- Narayan Iyer, Ph.D., Chief for Burn Medical Countermeasures, Biomedical Advanced Research and Development Authority, part of the Office of the Assistant Secretary for Preparedness and Response within the U.S. Department of Health and Human Services, Washington, D.C.
- Amanda Reichard, Ph.D., Project Officer, National Institute on Disability, Independent Living, and Rehabilitation Research, Washington, D.C.

The RAND team also extends its gratitude to the RAND Arlington, Virginia, office meeting support team, including Nina Ryan for project administrative assistance and Clara Aranibar, Jordan Bresnahan, Varun Chandorkar, Emily-Kate Chiusano, Carolyn Claybrooks, Katrina Doss-Owens, Silas Dustin, Sandra Facciolli, Gina Kalasky, Inez Khan, and Beth Seitzinger for notetaking support. Finally, the RAND team thanks Craig Bond, Emily Ward, and Jose Martinez for their thoughtful reviews.

Abbreviations

ABA	American Burn Association
ACB	*Acinetobacter calcoaceticus-baumannii*
ACS	American College of Surgeons
aKSs	autologous keratinocyte sheets
AP	action potential
AR	augmented reality
ASPR	Office of the Assistant Secretary for Preparedness and Response
BARDA	Biomedical Advanced Research and Development Authority
BICU	Burn Intensive Care Unit
BIPSR	Blast Injury Prevention Standards Recommendation
BIRCO	Blast Injury Research Coordinating Office
BW	body weight
CBRN	Chemical, Biological, Radiological, and Nuclear
CDC	Centers for Disease Control and Prevention
CNS	central nervous system
COTS	commercial-off-the-shelf
CRRT	continuous renal replacement therapy
CS	compartment syndrome
cTMS	combination thermosensitive
D	dextrorotatory
DHS	U.S. Department of Homeland Security
DoD	U.S. Department of Defense
ECM	extracellular matrix
ECMO	extracorporeal membrane oxygenation
EPO	erythropoietin
EPOR	erythropoietin receptors
FDA	U.S. Food and Drug Administration

FLE	fluorescent light energy
HSPC	Human Subjects Protection Committee
ICU	intensive care unit
IED	improvised explosive device
ISS	injury severity score
IV	intravenous
L	levorotatory
MC4R	melanocortin-4 receptor
MCM	medical countermeasure
MHS	military health system
MIC	minimum inhibitory concentration
NAC	N-acetyl-L-cysteine
NIDILRR	National Institute on Disability, Independent Living, and Rehabilitation Research
NIH	National Institutes of Health
OEF	Operation Enduring Freedom
OIF	Operation Iraqi Freedom
OTFC	oral transmucosal fentanyl citrate
PFC	prolonged field care
PTSD	posttraumatic stress disorder
QMAC	Quick Magnetic Analgesia Cuff
SoSM	State-of-the-Science Meeting
TBI	traumatic brain injury
TBSA	total body surface area
USAISR	U.S. Army Institute of Surgical Research
VA	U.S. Department of Veterans Affairs
WT	wild-type

CHAPTER ONE

State-of-the-Science Meeting Content Summary

The theme of the Ninth Department of Defense International State-of-the-Science Meeting (SoSM) on Blast Injury Research was "Mitigating the Effects of Blast-Related Burn Injuries from Prolonged Field Care to Rehabilitation and Resilience." The meeting was held from March 3 to March 5, 2020, at the RAND Corporation office in Arlington, Virginia, and more than 120 scientists, clinicians, and military leaders provided scientific overviews, presentations, and posters describing new and emerging science in the field. Before the meeting, a conference planning committee consulted on the literature review and research questions and served as a peer review panel for submitted abstracts, presentations, and posters. Six leading scientists and clinicians in related fields were invited to serve on an expert panel to lead working groups and develop overall recommendations.

The proceedings and findings from the meeting were intended to help answer the following questions:

1. What is the true scale and prevalence of blast-related burn injuries? What research is needed to better characterize the magnitude of this problem?
2. What skills, capabilities, and equipment are needed to better manage blast-related burns in the prolonged field care setting?
3. What are the most promising preventive and rehabilitative interventions for patients with blast-related burn injuries? What research is needed to understand the effectiveness and limitations of these interventions?
4. What are the most important gaps in research pertaining to blast-related burn injuries?

These conference proceedings provide summary information on (1) the background of the meeting, including working group findings, future directions, and recommendations; (2) the literature review that RAND researchers completed in support of the meeting; (3) the SoSM keynote address; and (4) all meeting presentations and abstracts. Supporting appendixes provide a list of previous SoSMs (Appendix A), the agenda for the SoSM (Appendix B), a biography of the keynote speaker (Appendix C), biographies of the expert panelists (Appendix D), and a list of the planning committee members (Appendix E). These proceedings will be of particular interest to scientists, clinicians, military personnel, and policymakers working in areas related to military medicine and health, blast injuries, and, of course, burn injury.

Background on Burn Injury

Blasts are complex events that can lead to multiple types of injuries through various mechanisms. Researchers tend to classify blast injuries into four (sometimes five) categories: primary injuries, caused by interactions between the blast wave and the body; secondary injuries, caused by debris carried by the blast; tertiary injuries, caused by physical displacement as a result of the pressure from the blast; and quaternary injuries, caused by secondary consequences of the blast, including thermal burns (Greer et al., 2016; Singh et al., 2016). Burn-relevant quinary effects can include infections of burn wounds, as well as bacterial, chemical, and radiological contamination (Cancio et al., 2017; Popivanov et al., 2014).

Compared with civilians, deployed service members are twice as likely to suffer a burn injury. Approximately 5 to 20 percent of combat-related casualties during Operation Iraqi Freedom (OIF) and Operation Enduring Freedom (OEF) included severe burns (Nuutila et al., 2019; Wolf, 2006), and burns constitute 10 percent of all combat-related injuries to the head and neck regions (Johnson et al., 2015). Observational research conducted between 2009 and 2011 in Afghanistan suggests that improvised explosive devices (IEDs) accounted for as much as 87 percent of all burns (Lairet et al., 2012). IED-related burns are at elevated risk of infection because they are often contaminated with dirt and debris (Murray, 2008). This is consistent with research that shows that burn injuries resulting from military operations are clinically different from burn injuries sustained by civilians given that service members are more likely to die of infection and gastrointestinal complications (Gomez et al., 2009). Infection control is essential for burn management because pathogens to which service members are exposed in current combat operations are increasingly resistant to antibiotics (Barillo, Pozza, and Margaret-Brandt, 2014). However, immediate evacuation might not always be possible. In these cases, burn injuries must be managed in a *prolonged field care* environment—i.e., field medical care is applied beyond doctrinal planning timelines until the patient can be delivered to definitive care—which presents challenges unique to military populations.

Working Group Questions, Answers, and Recommendations

Meeting attendees participated in one of five separate working groups, each led by one of the meeting expert panelists (listed in Appendix D). Initial questions were proposed by the RAND research team with input from the planning committee (listed in Appendix E). Working group responses were informed by members' own professional experiences and the groups' collective experiences, presentations, and posters.

Each working group was assigned a recorder, who organized discussion content and developed briefing materials in consultation with the expert panelist. At the end of the working group discussion period, each expert panelist presented the results of his or her group's discussion to all SoSM attendees. The findings from each working group were ultimately used to develop a list of key findings and recommendations from the SoSM. This section provides summaries of the responses developed by the working groups.

What Is the True Scale and Prevalence of Blast-Related Burn Injuries? What Research Is Needed to Better Characterize the Magnitude of This Problem?

Working groups noted that the nature of war is evolving and, with it, the type and severity of injuries. Blast and burn injuries are inherently complex and unique, requiring a multidisciplinary, team-oriented approach and extensive coordination between clinicians, researchers, scientists, and patients. Unfortunately, the true prevalence of blast-related burn injuries and the magnitude of this problem remain unknown, for a multitude of reasons—specifically, the fact that some data-collection and data-analysis tools are sorely lacking, and others are not being used or combined effectively. For example, such tools as Joint Trauma Analysis and Prevention of Injury in Combat should be leveraged to intersect the data silos and promote retrospective analyses of blast-related burn injuries. Marrying forensic data with clinical data also has the potential to clarify the effects of specific blast injuries on clinical outcomes.

Working groups emphasized that collaboration is paramount and should be conducted with a global perspective that goes beyond the individual level (e.g., patient, service member). *Global* is meant to include the U.S. Department of Defense (DoD) in its entirety, other U.S. government agencies (e.g., the U.S. Department of Veterans Affairs [VA], the National Institutes of Health [NIH], the Centers for Disease Control and Prevention [CDC], the U.S. Department of Homeland Security [DHS]), academia, and industry. Channels should be both built and opened to foster collaboration between any and all entities touching the field of blast-related burn injury. Additionally, the U.S. military could benefit significantly by partnering with researchers in low-intensity conflict sites to better test implementation of interventions in poorly resourced environments.

Working group participants also noted that data should be standardized across all institutions that care for blast-injury patients. A data repository to ensure continuity of care could include the recommended data categories of preparedness, bystander care, prehospital care, hospital care, rehabilitation, recovery, and community recovery and monitoring. Additionally, it is necessary to identify and standardize the most effective parameters for assessing, diagnosing, and treating blast-related burn injury, prior to the next conflict. For example, the injury severity score (ISS) is not specific enough for blast, burn, or inhalation injuries. Working group participants noted the need to develop a tool for assessing total body surface area (TBSA) that is more specific and takes into account location with respect to grading burn severity, along with potential rehabilitation needs. In addition, clinical documentation of injuries might need to be reexamined because of the fact that, dependent on the patient's circumstance and the number of International Classification of Diseases, Tenth Revision codes that could be documented, some injuries (such as burns) might not be captured in the records.

Once researchers can accurately identify how many patients are surviving a specific conflict or injury scenario, they will need to focus on long-term quality of life for survivors. Meaningful functional status, wound care, and physiological monitoring need to be incorporated. Additionally, there are research gaps and product deficiencies related to modeling injury, triage, wound care, real-time decision-support tools for first responders, and tools to help determine return to duty or escalation of care.

What Skills, Capabilities, and Equipment Are Needed to Better Manage Blast-Related Burns in the Prolonged Field Care Setting?

Although patient management has made significant advances in recent years, there is still much work to be done in the prolonged field care setting. Essential technical skills for field medics include wound decontamination, wound covering, pain management, hemorrhage control, airway security, debridement, and assessment of wound depth. To extend the "golden hour"—i.e., the first hour after the occurrence of a traumatic injury (which is considered the most critical for successful emergency treatment)—medics need to concentrate on wound management and infection control, because wound infections can significantly increase mortality and morbidity. Working group participants also noted the need for mobile medical units because of the multidimensional aspect of operations.

Diagnosis and treatment of fungal infections and sepsis are critical, as is implementation of the next generation of non-opioid pain management. Additional considerations posed by the working groups included augmenting service member immune response prior to deployment, further investigating the role of biomarkers, looking into the use of decision-support tools to help medics determine which patients can be treated in the field and which patients need to be evacuated, and expanding the use of unmanned aerial vehicles to collect intelligence, deliver products, and potentially evacuate patients.

Another critical aspect that the working groups discussed is increasing basic clinical skills and knowledge to prepare for the absence of technology in a near-peer combat setting. Additionally, working group participants noted that the prolonged field care setting often increases mental burden because of extended time frames. Further research should be conducted to determine the impact of triage and prolonged field care on troop morale, what the warfighter expects from medical personnel, the potential psychological impact of mis-triaging soldiers, and the increased cognitive load of using additional instruments and techniques.

As additional products are developed, it is important to evaluate whether these products limit mobility and increase the burden on service members as they carry individual first-aid kits or other products in the field. Additionally, experts emphasized the importance of incorporating enhancements into the mission-essential task list, a list of tasks that a unit must accomplish in combat.

What Are the Most Promising Preventive and Rehabilitative Interventions for Patients with Blast-Related Burn Injuries? What Research Is Needed to Understand the Effectiveness and Limitations of These Interventions?

Given the prevalence and severity of infections for blast-related burn injuries, the working group participants recommended focusing significant research efforts on understanding the challenge that infections pose, particularly fungal infections, and potential interventions. The most promising product in the treatment of burn injuries is a universal bandage. This would help reduce both the physical and mental burdens placed on medics from having to carry multiple targeted products that require highly specific injury assessment in the prolonged field care setting. Additionally, working group participants discussed the need to develop items or devices that can prevent injury, such as fire-retardant suits, and the need to conduct further research examining the efficacy of hemostatic agents to minimize the risk of hemorrhage (e.g., foam, drugs).

Research to assess the long-term consequences of blast-related burn injuries and the effectiveness of interventions is sorely needed, as is research to address how much rehabilitation is necessary, at what point, and whether there are sufficient staff to manage the patient load. To assess specific surgical restoration and reconstruction advances, the working group participants recommended multicenter clinical trials in both military and civilian hospitals.

In a separate vein, it is widely known that reproducible and translatable models are needed to better understand the effectiveness and limitations of interventions and advances, but such models for polytrauma currently do not exist. Participants agreed that it would be practical to start with simple models for fundamental changes induced by blast injury and, in time, build increasingly larger preclinical models until a human model is ready. Study designs are challenged by the stark differences in standards of care between a prolonged field care setting and a hospital setting. Clinical trials in this area are logistically difficult to conduct, so new settings or methods will need to be explored.

What Are the Most Important Gaps in Research Pertaining to Blast-Related Burn Injuries?

One of the gaps that consistently came up in discussion was data. Data need to be collected and standardized across all levels of care, and they need to be openly accessible. The issue is not necessarily that researchers lack a useful tool, but rather that researchers lack access to data—specifically, to usable data of sufficient quality—to better understand the scope of blast-related burn injuries from the point of injury all the way to recovery, rehabilitation, and reintegration. To improve data collection across the continuum of care, the data-sharing enterprise between DoD and VA needs to be strengthened. The handoff from acute to chronic care management should be reinforced, and opportunities to understand functional recovery should be shared. A journey map that documents the steps in patients' care—from point of injury to definitive care—to educate and guide blast-burn injury survivors through the recovery process could benefit patients and providers alike.

Working group participants also emphasized the gap in continuous feedback between end users and scientists during the product development cycle. Additionally, participants noted that product development should be linked to a regulatory or commercial strategy starting early in the process.

Expert Panel Discussion of Research Questions and Recommendations

Following the SoSM, there was a closed session with the expert panel to develop final recommendations for future research and suggestions for policy priorities. Working from the literature review summarizing scientific literature on blast-related burns, the SoSM presentations, and the working group findings, the expert panel developed final conference findings with proposed directions for future research. The RAND team took notes during the closed session, held on March 5, 2020, at the RAND office in Arlington, and subsequently synthesized them to create Table 1.1.

The following are overarching, high-level recommendations from the expert panel. For a list of expert panel members, see Appendix D.

Revisit Injury Classification and Data Collection Methods to Develop an Agreed-Upon Definition of *Blast-Related Burn Injuries* That Can Be Broadly Disseminated

The long-relied-upon ISS is not accurate enough to capture the effects of blast-related burn injuries. Successful polytrauma diagnosis and treatment require partnerships across medical specialties, from emergency medicine to rehabilitation, yet existing systems do not enable information-sharing across the continuum of care or between DoD, VA, and civilian health care systems. Furthermore, existing injury registries limit the ability to understand differences

Table 1.1
Research Questions and Recommendations by Domain

Domain	Research Questions and Recommendations
Bench research	Increase research on biomarkers, cytokines, and growth factors to improve wound care and treatment.
	Conduct a study of DNA biorepository and linkages to susceptibility and fitness.
Modeling development	Develop a combined blast-injury model.
	Develop a model for product development.
Classification, common data elements, and data collection	Evaluate the need for a new classification system for burns that incorporates TBSA, method of injury, location of injury, rehabilitation needs, etc.
	Evaluate existing data collection efforts to understand differences across collection methods and improve data quality.
	What is the best way to facilitate data collection, comparison, and collaboration with civilian trauma communities?
	What is the best way to organize data collection? What technology products would facilitate data collection?
Coordination and collaboration	What systems exist for active military, veterans, and civilian clinicians and scientists to collaborate?
	Develop tabletop exercises for an influx of blast-related burn patients on a nationwide basis to fully stress the system, expose weaknesses, and involve all of the actors most likely to be involved.
	Provide a continuum of care from a forward-deployed setting through the military and veteran health systems.
Global health engagement	What opportunities does global health engagement provide to enhance a ready medical force, and how would DoD harness these opportunities?
Quality improvement	Does provider training and feedback improve appropriate response to burn wounds?
	Codify After Action Reports and other past responses to preserve institutional memory of wound care from prolonged field care, rehabilitation, and resilience.
	Document best practices for transitions of care from point of care to reintegration.
Ready medical providers	Do gaps exist between the current state of training and future needs?
	How are burn casualties of future conflicts likely to differ from those of previous conflicts, and how will these differences affect medical treatment? How do those treatment needs translate into requirements that providers must meet to be considered ready for future deployments?
	Develop an evidence-informed framework for defining a ready medical provider for wartime burn care.
	Develop decision frameworks for burn assessments and evacuation guidelines.
	Develop a "stop the burn" training module.
	Assess providing universal medical training for burn wound care for all forward-facing personnel.
	Develop educational modules on local medical practices (i.e., practices to consider and aspects to reject).
Telehealth	What is the feasibility of virtual health care delivery over large distances using telehealth? What are the potential limitations of this approach?
	What is the feasibility of empowering service members to provide self-care and buddy care?
	Increase research on understanding cognitive burden in the use of telehealth and telecommunication for patient management.

Table 1.1—Continued

Domain	Research Questions and Recommendations
Technology	Evaluate virtual training platforms for clinicians that reduce training time and improve performance.
	Evaluate technology-assisted rehabilitation programs to enhance inpatient programs or compliance with daily exercise and the impact on psychological recovery.
	Where is there a need for artificial intelligence, machine learning, and other emerging technologies that have multiuse applications to support wound care?
	Incentivize synergy for joint product development.
	Incentivize discovery of innovative products for wound care and infection prevention, preventative products (e.g., flame-retardant uniforms), products that can arrest burn conversion, portable ventilators, non-opioid treatment for pain management, and next-generation dressings.
	Incentivize development of *theranostics*—i.e., devices that treat and diagnose (e.g., smart bandages).
	Develop a requirements process that is nimble, is process- and solutions-driven, and has continuous user feedback.
	Develop decision-support tools.
	Develop non-intravenous (non-IV) resuscitation strategies.
	Increase research on immune response, metabolism, anabolic agents, and topical agents to protect against radiation or chemical burns.

in interventions and outcomes. A critical gap is the near-absence of completed prospective longitudinal studies with follow-up longer than one year.

The many aspects of burn injury, including TBSA, method of injury, location of injury, polytrauma, and rehabilitation needs, should be incorporated into data repositories. Once parameters are defined, existing data collection methods should be evaluated, and the ideal methods to facilitate comparison and collaboration with civilian trauma communities should be codified into clinical practice guidelines. This can be accomplished by first developing an agreed-upon definition of *blast-related burn injuries* and then broadly disseminating it for consistent use.

Develop Improved Training and Guidance to Support Burn-Injury Management in Prolonged Field Care Settings

Focusing on accelerating the pathway from knowledge acquisition to new-and-improved training of forward service members is crucial to meet their needs in current and future conflicts. A set of agreed-upon knowledge, skills, and abilities should be incorporated into revised training curricula for field medics, clinicians, and service members trained in buddy care. More specifically, to decrease morbidity and mortality, medics need to be able to prevent burn wound conversion, avert infections, and manage common comorbidities, such as fluid loss, organ damage, and other afflictions associated with blasts. Once service members are evacuated, military and civilian trauma units must have both the capacity and the training necessary to provide higher levels of care.

Strengthen Rehabilitation Practices to Enhance Continuity of Care and Emphasize a Return to Full Function

The most underdeveloped area of empirical research that the RAND team reviewed pertained to rehabilitative approaches for blast-injured patients with severe burn injuries. Physical, occupational, and psychosocial rehabilitation should begin as soon as possible after injury and should be viewed as a lifelong task to reduce pain, improve range of motion, and strengthen both the physical and psychological abilities to resume daily life. Technology-assisted rehabilitation programs can enhance inpatient programs, improve compliance with daily regimes, and have positive impacts on resilience. Best practices for the various transitions from point of care through rehabilitation should be developed and widely disseminated to civilian, military, and VA facilities.

Conduct Additional Research on Burn Management in Theater

Experts noted that many treatments and products employed in the field are decades old. Although promising new products and approaches have been identified, further testing (involving computational models, animal models, and clinical trials) is needed. Researchers should investigate topical products to arrest burn conversion, theranostics to diagnose and treat injuries, and non-IV resuscitation strategies and should conduct basic research on immune response, biomarkers, metabolic impacts, and anabolic agents. Product development should focus on portability, durability, and stability in theater, as well as flexibility in terms of application for multiple wounds. Computer and large-animal models should be used to test treatments of burn injuries caused by the next generation of weapons.

CHAPTER TWO

Literature Review Summary

The U.S. Army Medical Research and Development Command and the DoD Blast Injury Research Coordinating Office (BIRCO) sponsored the ninth SoSM for blast injury research to identify what is known and not known regarding key blast injury–related topics and emerging issues. The topic of the SoSM was "Mitigating the Effects of Blast-Related Burn Injuries from Prolonged Field Care to Rehabilitation and Resilience." To inform the SoSM and the associated work group and recommendation process, the BIRCO requested that the RAND National Defense Research Institute conduct a comprehensive literature review on burn injury following blast injury. (For details, see Engel et al., 2020.)

The RAND research team, in collaboration with the planning committee, developed four main literature review objectives:

1. Describe the epidemiology and outcomes of blast-related burn injury.
2. Review the evidence on prevention and acute management of blast-related burn injuries.
3. Review the evidence on prolonged field care for blast-related burn injuries.
4. Review the evidence on and innovations related to chronic care of blast-related burn injuries.

To complete this review of articles from 2008 to 2019, RAND researchers defined key research questions about blast-related and military-relevant burns, identified articles meeting a defined set of inclusion criteria in the peer-reviewed scientific literature and the DoD grey literature, documented and coded key article features, and synthesized and analyzed the abstracted data. Article findings were synthesized using the continuum of health research, from foundational research to health services research, as defined in the National Research Action Plan, outlined by DoD and VA. Articles written in a language other than English were excluded, as were articles not in the public domain (e.g., classified, For Official Use Only).

Results of the Literature Review

Among identified articles, basic and applied clinical research had roughly equal representation. The body of the literature review further summarizes the studies on the biophysiological mechanisms of blast-related burn injuries and complications, the incidence and prevalence of burn injuries, and aspects of acute and long-term burn care.

Future Research Directions from the Literature Review and Synthesis of the Evidence

The following suggestions for further research are based on the results of the literature review and synthesis of the evidence. (Final recommendations from the expert panel are provided in Chapter One.)

Invest in Research Areas Where the Epidemiology Indicates a Greater Need for Improvement in Clinical Care and Service Delivery

The epidemiological literature provides a direct indication of the most frequent comorbidities, sequelae, and causes of mortality associated with burn-related injury. Therefore, it would be valuable to map these findings onto the existing treatment research portfolio to identify areas that are understudied and underinvested. Studies addressing prevention and treatment of infection, as well as inhalation injury, are critical to better address burn injury and would be particularly valuable in the prolonged field care setting, where access to antiseptics and other resources is restricted.

Prevention efforts likewise require additional research. Overall, additional research measuring the relative value of investments in prevention versus treatment could have significant value and generate cost savings. There is limited research on prevention of blast-related burns, including only a small set of informational campaigns that could be implemented in a military context. Additionally, research testing the application of current diagnostic and severity assessment tools in military contexts would be valuable.

Review How Guidelines Are Developed, How Often They Are Updated, and How the Guidelines Integrate New Evidence

The RAND team found a significant number of systematic literature reviews pertaining to blast-related burn injuries. However, the synthesis of these into a systematic and routinely updated set of guidelines appears to be lacking. The RAND team recommends updating burn-injury care guidelines at regular intervals to account for evolving best practices and innovations.

Expand Research Specifically Addressing Prolonged Field Care for Blast-Related Burn Injuries

Few studies have addressed prolonged field care. The evolving nature of adversaries' capabilities, military operations, and weaponry suggests that prolonged field care capabilities are essential for managing severe blast-related burns. The literature has outlined several areas requiring further research, including the impact of training clinicians in forward treatment of blast-related burns on outcomes, improved training in fluid resuscitation and pain management, and the design and subsequent dissemination of forward burn kits. Meanwhile, researchers are gaining momentum in the biosynthetic wound management product space, and the research seems promising. However, studies have been small, and applicability to prolonged field care remains to be proven. Finally, there remains plenty of space for further research studies that yield direct applications for use in the prolonged field care setting, such as silver-nylon dressings that are uniquely portable, are easy to use, and possess key antimicrobial properties.

Develop Enhanced Care Coordination and Triage Strategies for Civilian Burn Patients Receiving Care in Military Treatment Facilities

International humanitarian law states that emergency medical support must be provided for civilians, including children, who are injured in conflicts. However, there is limited research on triage algorithms and systematic emergency-treatment guidelines for civilian burn patients receiving care at military treatment facilities in combat areas. Providing forward treatment for civilians with noncombat burn injuries at field hospitals can have a significant impact on facility operations, including bed space, operating room supplies, and nursing time. Furthermore, the availability of surgery to treat burn injuries and technology to perform skin grafting is uncommon in local civilian treatment facilities in combat areas, which creates difficulty in planning discharge and follow-up care for civilian burn patients who need significant aftercare. Although there are extensive protocols for evacuating military members who sustain serious burn injuries to higher-level facilities, civilian patients are presented with fewer opportunities for comprehensive emergency burn care and effective aftercare delivered locally, thereby increasing the likelihood of poor outcomes. Emergency department triage algorithms for use in civilian mass casualty incidents involving burns should be modified and tested for the military setting.

CHAPTER THREE

Keynote Address

COL Kevin K. Chung, M.D., delivered the keynote address to attendees of the ninth SoSM. Chung, a graduate of the U.S. Military Academy at West Point and Georgetown University School of Medicine, is currently chair of the Department of Medicine at the Uniformed Services University of the Health Sciences in Bethesda, Maryland. Previously, he was chief of medicine at Brooke Army Medical Center at Fort Sam Houston, Texas. He also served at the U.S. Army Institute of Surgical Research (USAISR), where he was medical director of the Burn Intensive Care Unit (BICU), Task Area Manager of Clinical Trials in Burns and Trauma, and director of research for the research directorate.

During his keynote, Chung discussed major technological advances that occur during wartime. Fear of failure can paralyze progress; however, the urgency of war dispels this fear, thereby accelerating progress. One example of such an advance was bringing extracorporeal membrane oxygenation (ECMO) to the field. The introduction of ECMO facilitated in-theater treatment of steam inhalation injuries and full thickness airway burns by continuous renal replacement therapy (CRRT) nurses. The subsequent introduction of renal replacement therapy in theater helped address acute kidney injury.

Chung then spoke about the next generation of field medical advances, discussing how each and every advance resulted in increased survivability for the sickest of patients. He urged the group to remember that all interventions are justified in the hope of a meaningful recovery.

CHAPTER FOUR

Invited Speaker Presentation Summaries

This chapter provides summaries of the invited speaker presentations, written from notes we took during the SoSM.

Blast-Related Burns: A Modern History

Leopoldo (Lee) C. Cancio, M.D. (U.S. Army Burn Center, USAISR), opened the scientific meeting with a chronicle of treating blast-related burns from World War I to the present day. This history emphasized the need for risk-taking innovations to advance biomedical progress. Each improvement should be rapidly published and disseminated. Cancio estimated that, depending on the conflict, significant burns complicated approximately 5 to 10 percent of combat casualties. Furthermore, he remarked that there is a supply-demand mismatch with respect to resources and skills. Most deployed providers have minimal burn experience prior to deployment, leaving them ill-prepared for the complicated injury patterns and resuscitation demands presented by blast-related burns. Cancio argued that future battlefields will require a focus on triage for prolonged field care. Leaders will need to consider whether strategic aeromedical evacuation is available and which patients are stable enough, with sufficient resources, for transport to an intensive care unit (ICU) to be postponed. During the planning phase for OIF, the possibility of a large number of burn patients, exceeding the capacity of USAISR, was considered. Although this scenario did not materialize, it emphasizes the need for a networked system connecting burn centers across the United States that can accept surplus patients and train providers in the most up-to-date techniques, particularly in light of a possible future conflict with a near-peer adversary.

Overview of DoD Burn Research

Kai Leung, M.D. (USAISR), provided a broad overview of the state of burn-injury research in the context of multidomain operations and prolonged field care. This focus is driven by senior military leadership's anticipation of peer-to-peer conflict where multiple complementary large-scale threats are integrated across domains with limited evacuation options. There are numerous tactical problems associated with prolonged care in multidomain operations, many of which have fatal outcomes, such as infection, septic shock, compartment syndrome, and prolonged pain and delirium. To improve survivability and reduce morbidity, the DoD research program seeks to optimize burn resuscitation, decrease local and systemic inflammation, and fabricate dressings to limit progression and complication of burn wounds. The DoD research program emphasizes innovations in triage, resuscitation, wound coverage, and wound debridement. Leung further described the Army's strategic plan end-state goals for handling severe burns while maintaining warfighter lethality:

- **End-State Goal 1:** Provide capability and capacity to accurately assess burn injuries, enabling expeditionary medical providers at the point of need to sustain warfighter and unit lethality.
- **End-State Goal 2:** Accelerate service member return to duty following a severe burn in the operational environment to preserve the fighting force and minimize morbidity in burn casualties normally requiring evacuation.
- **End-State Goal 3:** Provide effective initial in-theater treatments for 100 percent of warfighters with severe or disabling burn injuries to improve recovery and minimize morbidity and mortality.
- **End-State Goal 4:** Provide advanced treatments for life-threatening or disabling burn sequelae to minimize mortality and morbidity secondary to severe burns.

Several additional solutions were proposed to support the prolonged field care setting, such as a wound dressing with silver nitrate to temporize the wound; field-deployable devices for assessing burn severity and TBSA, performing nonsurgical debridement, and guiding fluid resuscitation; and treatments to prevent burn wound progression and conversion.

Military Health System Burn Injury Prevention Standard: Example of Dermal Burn Science

Jeffrey Colombe, Ph.D. (MITRE Corporation), offered an overview of the science of burn injury and its effect on the skin. He spoke about the Blast Injury Prevention Standards Recommendation (BIPSR) process that is undergoing an evaluation over 14 body regions. Candidate standards support health hazard assessments for the medical community and survivability assessments. Colombe described the dermal burn classification system and the effects of the patient's increased burn severity on that individual's physical and system-level health outcomes. Additionally, he emphasized that severe burns can lead to immunosuppression, which can lead to infections outside the burn site, or a months-long hypermetabolic state, which can lead to decreased bone density, muscle weakness, and improper healing of burns and other wounds.

Civilian Burn Mass Casualty Events and Preparedness Research

Colleen Ryan, M.D. (Harvard Medical School), shared what the military health system can learn from the civilian sector and how both systems could work together to support surge capacity. She stated that burn care is no longer in the surgical training curriculum, and there are only 1,800 burn care beds spread across the country. After summarizing recent advances in surgical reconstruction techniques, Ryan explained that lessons learned tend to be qualitative assessments; however, if something can be measured, it can be improved. Applied convergence science, or the integration of knowledge, tools, and thought strategies, can help develop crisis standards of care. These standards of care guide evidence-based tools for triage that are ethical, proportional, and accountable, and require a full assessment with a performance improvement process. Finally, Ryan shared that the American Burn Association (ABA) burn triage tables have been tested in emergency exercises but need to be electronically automated for ready access in a crisis. Exercises emphasized the need for shared learning between burn centers, telemedicine consultations, and stronger networks and coordination to address the needs of excess patients.

Prehospital Burn Care: Prolonged Field Care

COL Jeremy Pamplin, M.D. (Telemedicine and Advanced Technology Research Center, U.S. Army Medical Research and Development Command), defined and discussed research gaps in prolonged field care for burns. Pamplin defined *prolonged field care* as "field medical care, applied beyond doctrinal planning time-lines, in order to decrease patient mortality and morbidity. It utilizes limited resources and is sustained until the patient arrives at an appropriate level of care." He emphasized that prolonged field care is not the operational plan but should be anticipated and planned for. Austere medicine is characterized by limited resources of equipment, medicine, diagnostics, personnel, knowledge, skills, abilities, and expertise. A review of 54 prolonged field care cases identified a set of ideal skill sets, listed in Table 4.1.

In addition, Pamplin identified ten capabilities that combine basic diagnostic and patient treatment skills with medical equipment: monitor the patient; resuscitate the patient; ventilate or oxygenate; maintain an airway; sedate or control pain; perform a physical exam; provide nursing, hygiene, and comfort measures; perform advanced surgical interventions; conduct telemedicine; and prepare the patient for flight. Pamplin estimated that engagements in austere environments could postpone evacuation to a critical care facility by one to three days. Pamplin recommended that, to be better prepared, stakeholders should implement a telemedicine system for routine, urgent, and emergent care; develop better TBSA assessments; develop

Table 4.1
Identified Prolonged Field Care Skill Sets

Area	Description
Simple interventions	Measuring serial vital signs
	Measuring urine output
	Interpreting trends over time
Complex interventions	Prolonged mechanical ventilation and airway management
	Sedation and analgesia pressor and fluid management
Procedures	Tube thoracostomy
	Cricothyroidotomy
	Fasciotomy
	Escharotomy
Telemedicine	Assistance where there are knowledge and experience gaps

SOURCE: Jeremy Pamplin, ninth SoSM presentation.

better alternative topical agents and the next generation of IV fluids; and improve resuscitation techniques. Finally, he suggested that models should reflect the austere environment in which service members will be located.

Acute Assessment and Management of Burn Injury

Eileen Bulger, M.D. (University of Washington), spoke on the complex polytrauma challenges posed by blast injuries. Assessing these injuries should start with *ABC*—airway, breathing, and circulation—followed by diagnosis of traumatic brain injury (TBI) and other injuries difficult to diagnose in a prehospital setting. Bulger emphasized that addressing hypothermia is critical in a prolonged field care scenario because blood will not clot when cold. For better management of future blast-induced polytrauma, Bulger recommended (1) determining the optimal approach to fluid resuscitation (she cautioned against administering too much fluid), (2) managing blast lung and inhalation injuries, and (3) providing optimal excision care and wound management. In the long term, technology that can stop internal hemorrhage without a surgeon would benefit response to civilian and military traumas. The system is significantly challenged by the regionalization of care in combined Level 1 trauma burn centers and the lack of familiarity with mass casualty events. In moments of crisis, providers might be distracted by burn injuries and overlook life-threatening secondary injuries. In the absence of a larger network of providers, just-in-time training and telemedicine can supplement training.

Impact of Acute Care on Long Term Outcomes

Nicole S. Gibran, M.D. (University of Washington), argued that a burn is not an episodic event, but rather a continuous challenge that should be classified as a chronic condition. Improved survival rates, attributable to improved care, are illustrated in Figure 4.1. A historical analysis of the National Trauma Database E-Codes found that most burn injuries associated with an explosion were isolated burns that resulted in low mortality (3.7 percent), which reinforces the need to look at long-term care. There is an indirect relationship between complications and quality of life; the Short Form Health Survey (SF-12) physical component score doubles after three complications. In inhalation injuries specifically, physical component scores are poor predictors of quality of life. The transition from zero preventable deaths to zero preventable disabilities should include examination of how hypertrophic scars, contraction, pigmentation, Marjolijn ulcers, and itching are tied to disability.

Surgical Advances: Reconstruction and Restoration

Rodney Chan, M.D., and MAJ Julie Rizzo (U.S. Army Institute for Surgical Research), shared several recent case studies of plastic and reconstructive surgery. They emphasized that reconstruction should start early, with key stakeholders involved as early in the process as possible. Stakeholders include surgeons and experts in orthopedics, prosthetics, rehabilitation, and behavioral health. To provide durable vascularized soft-tissue coverage, surgeons should (1) protect wounds (e.g., keep the wound sealed using vacuum-assisted closure), (2) maintain moisture on wound surfaces, and (3) protect extremities for later procedures, such as attaching prostheses. Additional principles are recommended in Table 4.2.

Chan and Rizzo emphasized the importance of team approaches to polytrauma and concluded by asserting that, even in prolonged field care scenarios, "a general surgeon is just a trauma surgeon downrange."

Figure 4.1
Increased Survival from Acute Burns

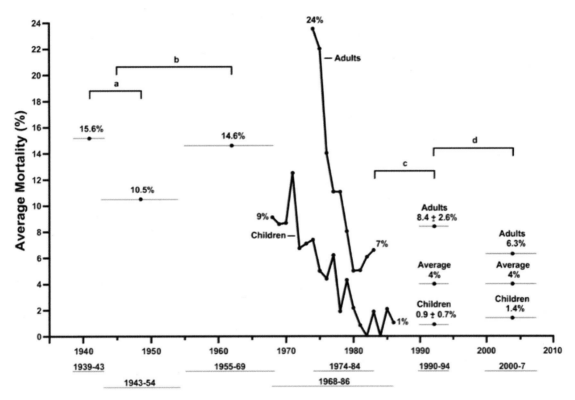

SOURCE: Ronald G. Tompkins, "Survival from Burns in the New Millennium: 70 Years' Experience from a Single Institution," *Annals of Surgery*, Vol. 261, No. 2, February 2015, pp. 263–268. Used with permission.

Table 4.2
Reconstruction Principles After Blast Injury

Stage of Treatment	Reconstruction Recommendation
Early	Perform aggressive debridement to control contamination.
	Preserve viable tissue by meticulous and careful dissection and early coverage of vital structures (e.g., viscera, bones, tendons).
	Delay complex reconstruction until after the acute phase.
Late	Focus on preserving and maximizing function and minimizing donor morbidity.
	Improve skin quality at the interfaces with prosthetics; anticipate prolonged pressure while sitting or standing in this patient population.

SOURCE: Rodney Chan and Julie Rizzo, ninth SoSM presentation.

Psychosocial Aspects of Resilience and Functioning

Amanda Reichard, Ph.D. (National Institute on Disability, Independent Living, and Rehabilitation Research [NIDILRR]), spoke on factors contributing to resilience and long-term functioning in injured soldiers. The American Psychological Association defines *resilience* as "the process of adapting well in the face of adversity, trauma, tragedy, threats, or significant sources of stress. As much as resilience involves 'bouncing back' from these difficult experiences, it can also involve profound personal growth" (Palmiter et al., 2012). Reichard said that contributing factors to learned resilience are positive relationships, self-image, good communication skills, problem-solving, and social networks. Burn-injury recovery is a complex, ongoing, biopsychosocial process in which physical and mental health are interrelated. In addition to physical outcomes, burn patients can experience psychosocial outcomes, such as depression, posttraumatic stress disorder (PTSD), and anxiety; issues with body image and deformity; substance use disorders; and lack of social use disorders. Reichard said that burn injuries do not predict psychosocial outcomes, thus validating the need for early screening and psychological counseling. She warned that, because of the severity of blast-related burn injuries, psychological conditions can be overlooked, and reintegration can be delayed. Reichard concluded by saying that future research should involve the unique perspective of burn survivors and focus on the development and empirical testing of assessment tools and interventions.

CHAPTER FIVE

Scientific Presentation Summaries

In consultation with the planning committee, the RAND team selected abstracts to accept for oral presentations upon evaluation of the title and the abstract. This chapter provides summaries of the scientific presentations, written from notes that the RAND team took during the SoSM.

Burn Injuries in U.S. Service Members: 2001–2018

Katheryne Perez, M.P.H. (Naval Health Research Center), shared her team's analysis of the Expeditionary Medical Encounter Database, which contains all deployment-related injury data from point of injury through rehabilitation. Figure 5.1 demonstrates how, from 2001 through 2018, the incidence of burn injuries aligned with the intensity of OIF and OEF.

Perez noted that, unlike deployment-related amputations, which typically affect lower extremities, approximately one-third of burn-related amputations are in the upper extremities. Results from this study can be used to serve as a baseline for future research, inform planning

Figure 5.1
Service Members with Burn Injuries, by Year

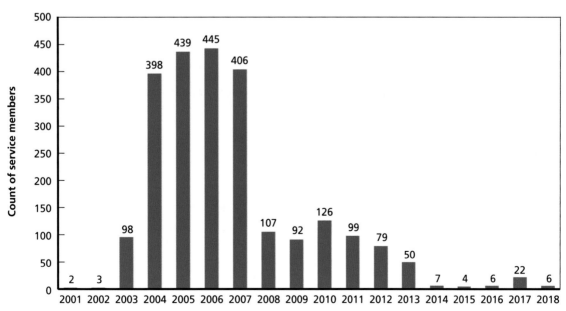

SOURCE: Katheryne Perez, ninth SoSM presentation.

and preparation of care, and aid in the development of new measures to prevent or mitigate the effects of blast injuries.

U.S. Army Burn Center Registry and Burn Injury Model System

Radha K. Holavanahalli, Ph.D. (University of Texas Southwestern Medical Center), presented collaborative research uses for the U.S. Army Burn Center registry and the civilian Burn Injury Model System. The goal of this effort is twofold: (1) to have a continuous and seamless exchange of knowledge between the sectors available for education, research, and training opportunities and (2) to facilitate a national strategic approach to long-term burn outcomes. Holavanahalli argued that, because burn survival rates have resulted in longer life spans, there needs to be a paradigm shift to increase focus on long-term outcomes and quality of life for survivors. The joint approach to study the continuum of burn trauma care is illustrated in Figure 5.2.

As DoD prepares for future conflicts, possibly without air superiority and with the need for prolonged field care, these data can help prioritize acute care and triage classification and improve the knowledge base regarding when service members can return to battle. Holavanahalli also shared the Burn Injury Model System's center program—one of three multicenter programs sponsored by NIDILRR to examine outcomes following the delivery of a coordinated system of acute trauma care and rehabilitation. The program studies the long-term physical, psychological, social, and vocational aspects of recovery. The ultimate goal is to package findings for different stakeholders in the form of fact sheets and multimedia presentations.

Figure 5.2
A Joint Approach to Burn Trauma Care Centered on Shared Aims and Common Standards

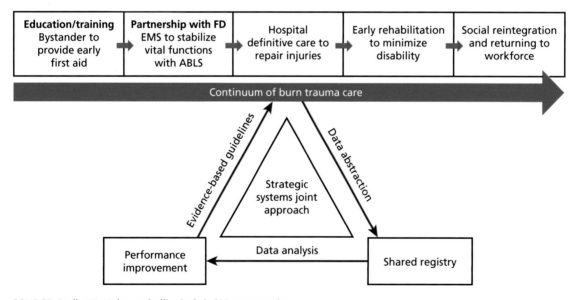

SOURCE: Radha K. Holavanahalli, ninth SoSM presentation.
NOTE: ABLS = Advanced Burn Life Support; EMS = emergency medical services; FD = fire department.

TBI, Burns and Blast: Is PTSD All About the Blast?

Mary Jo Pugh, Ph.D., RN (Informatics, Decision-Enhancement and Analytic Sciences Center, VA Salt Lake City), spoke about the comorbidities of burns, blasts, and TBIs. TBI combined with burn injury and non–central nervous system (non-CNS) trauma doubles mortality compared with burn with non-CNS trauma. Long-term outcomes of blast-related burn injuries, particularly in conjunction with TBI, suggest that PTSD is prevalent shortly after a blast injury, although little data exist on long-term outcomes for PTSD. Linking the DoD Trauma Registry and veterans' records, the team hypothesized that veterans with blast-induced TBIs and burn injuries would exhibit higher rates of PTSD than those with only blast injuries. The team found that soldiers suffering from blast injuries were more likely to be diagnosed with PTSD than those without, regardless of whether burn injuries were also present. Factors that lengthened the time to diagnosis were profound injuries as determined by ISS, officer versus enlisted status, and multiple deployments. Future studies with this data set will focus on the mechanism behind severe physical injuries being linked to higher incidences of PTSD.

National Trauma Research Action Plan: A Burn Research Agenda

Nicole S. Gibran, M.D. (University of Washington), described the 2016 National Academies of Sciences, Engineering, and Medicine (NASEM) report calling for a national integrated military-civilian trauma action plan to achieve zero preventable deaths and disabilities after injury. The NASEM report included a proposal to establish a National Trauma Research Action Plan to "strengthen trauma research and ensure that the resources available for this research are commensurate with the importance of injury and the potential for improvement in patient outcomes" (National Academies of Sciences, Engineering, and Medicine, 2016). To address this recommendation, the Coalition for National Trauma Research was funded by DoD to generate a comprehensive research agenda spanning the continuum of trauma and burn care from prehospital care to rehabilitation. The Burn group represented one of 11 focus areas for development of this research agenda.

Experts in burn care and research were identified and recruited to identify current gaps in clinical burn research, generate research questions, and establish the priority of these questions using a consensus-driven Delphi survey approach. Participants were identified using established Delphi recruitment guidelines to ensure heterogeneity and generalizability, and both military and civilian representatives were included. Literature reviews were conducted to inform the panel. Panelists were encouraged, but not required, to use a PICO format to generate research questions: Patient/population, Intervention, Compare/control, Outcome model. On subsequent surveys, participants were asked to rank the priority of each research question on a nine-point Likert scale, which was categorized to represent low-, medium-, and high-priority items. Consensus was defined based on more than 60 percent of panelists agreeing on the priority category. Thirty-eight burn subject-matter experts generated 959 questions in 14 key topic areas. After editing for duplication, 949 questions were included in the priority ranking. Although the topic areas included prehospital care and mass casualty burn disaster, no questions addressed blast injury specifically. By round 3 of the process, 395 questions (42 percent) reached 60-percent consensus. Of these, 252 (64 percent) were high, 101 (26 percent) medium, and 42 (11 percent) low priority. A summary of the high-priority questions that relate to burn care was presented. Many of the high-priority questions facing the clinical care of burn patients translate to issues faced in the setting of blast-burn injury. However, the absence of specific questions related to blast injuries highlights the gap in knowledge and need for prioritization of research related to burns caused by blast injury.

A Warrior Avatar for Model Based Blast and Burn Injury

H. T. Garimella, Ph.D. (CFD Research Group), summarized several human models for blast and burn injury currently in development. User-friendly software tools and mobile applications are needed for model-based personalized assessments and management of blast and burn injuries. In the future, human anatomy mesh models, high-fidelity photography, and reduced-order models could calculate TBSA for total cutaneous functional units. By better understanding injury mechanisms, researchers can design protective measures, diagnostics, and treatments. Additionally, Garimella argued that patients with smaller burns might not need to be evacuated—in fact, evacuation could worsen outcomes. A combination of risk-prediction tools and telemedicine might help inform evacuation decisions.

In Vivo Terahertz Spectral Imaging for Burn Depth Diagnosis

M. Hassan Arbab, Ph.D. (Stony Brook University), summarized recent progress in biomedical applications for spectral imaging. Historically, there has been a gap between electronics and photonics coverage—what Arbab coined the "terahertz gap," as shown in Figure 5.3. Different technologies use different parts of the electromagnetic spectrum, but few technologies use the terahertz frequency. Recent technological advances permit generation of up to 1 mW of power, which can be used for cancer imaging, single-contrast imaging (similar to magnetic resonance imaging), or burn imaging, or even by DHS to scan luggage. Next-stage developments will focus on a handheld spectral imager to compare spectral images for burn criteria, healing times, and burn types.

Figure 5.3
Terahertz Waves in the Electromagnetic Spectrum

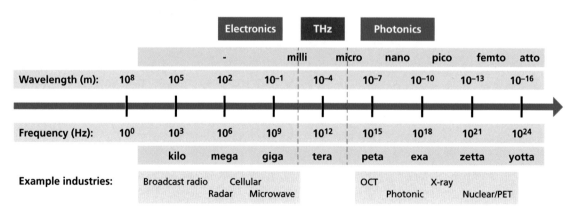

SOURCE: M. Hassan Arbab, ninth SoSM presentation.
NOTE: OCT = optical coherence tomography, PET = positron emission tomography; THz = terahertz.

Creating an Automated, Enhanced Lund Browder Diagram to Calculate TBSA

Gregory T. Rule, P.E. (Applied Research Associates, Inc.), emphasized the need for a method of estimating burn size that is less prone to error than human assessment. Estimating TBSA is necessary for the development of initial fluid-resuscitation and patient-management plans, yet assessing injuries in the field is frequently done by someone with limited to no experience with burns. If burn depths can be better estimated, particularly partial-thickness burns that are highly variable, severe outcomes could be mitigated. Rule and his colleagues developed a lightweight, portable, multispectral photography platform designed to function in austere environments. Using standardized pose templates common in clinical care, the team trained a machine learning algorithm to function in different ambient light conditions, identify body parts, and even differentiate clothing from skin. In time, the multi-speckle imaging (MSI) camera system might take the form of a camera that can attach to devices in the field, not unlike the Nett Warrior or the Microsoft HoloLens.

Blood mRNA Integrity Is a Marker of Radiation Exposure

Lauren Moffatt, Ph.D. (MedStar Health Research Institute), shared recent biomarker research used to differentiate thermal injuries from radiation burns and to determine the severity or extent of a burn. She noted that any biomarker candidates will need to be rapidly identifiable, reproducible in a broad population, reliable, and as noninvasive as possible. Earlier research found that data tended to cluster by the dose of radiation delivered. In murine studies, as the radiation dose increased, there was a significant drop in the quality of ribonucleic acid (RNA) integrity. The radiation dose had a stronger correlation with RNA integrity number values for blood than for skin. Research is ongoing on the impact of aging on biomarkers and sensitivity, a rapid assay or kit to guide early interventions, and field tests that can be used for polytrauma in military or civilian contexts.

Burn Resuscitation: Can We Be Better?

Jeanne Lee, M.D. (University of California, San Diego [UCSD] Health), described an effort to avoid over-resuscitation of burn patients. Since World War II, several formulas have been devised to estimate the fluid requirements for burn patients. The Evans and Brooke formulas used a combination of plasma and saline but were eventually abandoned because of the high rates of hepatitis transmission in poorly screened plasma. Today, most burn centers use a variation of the Parkland (Baxter) or modified Brooke formulas, which calculate volume, weight, and TBSA, and advocate delaying the use of albumin for 24 to 48 hours after injury. Clinicians recognized that under-resuscitation led to poor organ perfusion and renal failure; however, fluid creep became a problem, and patients received in excess of what the Parkland formulas predicted. Lee and colleagues hypothesized that, to avoid over-resuscitation and inconsistent implementation of resuscitation protocols, a nurse-driven protocol with early use of fresh frozen plasma would reduce the use of crystalloid fluids and potentially reduce the need for CRRT. They piloted a nurse-driven protocol based on urine output, outlined in Figure 5.4. Early findings confirmed the hypothesis and will be used to analyze UCSD resuscitation practices and continue to decrease the use of crystalloids and avoid the phenomenon of fluid creep.

Figure 5.4
Nurse-Driven Fluid-Resuscitation Clinical Pathway

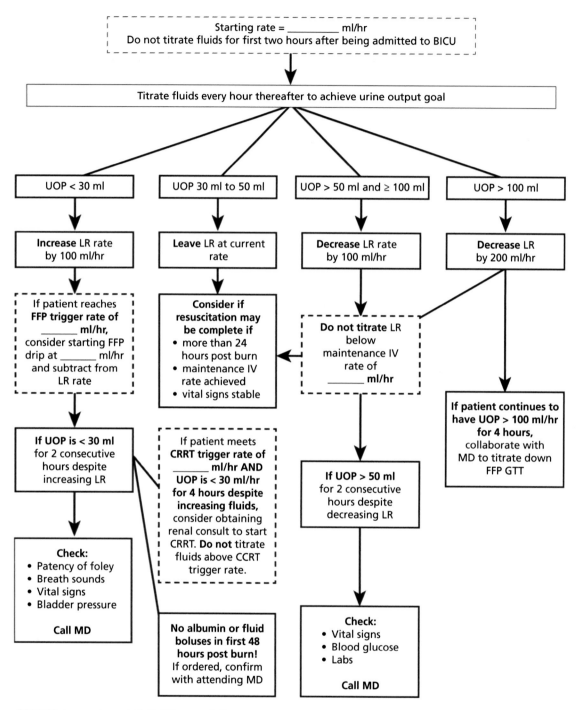

SOURCE: Jeanne Lee, ninth SoSM presentation.
NOTE: FFP = fresh frozen plasma; GTT = glucose tolerance test; LR = lactated Ringer's; MD = medical doctor; UOP = urine output.

Nanofiber Dressings for Infection Prevention and Pain Relief

Jessica Amber Jennings, Ph.D. (University of Memphis), shared recent advances in burn dressings to enhance coverage, prevent infection, and minimize pain. Traditional antibiotics are unable to sufficiently address bacteria within biofilm that forms on burn tissues. Several molecules, such as cis-2-deceonic acid, work with antimicrobials to disperse biofilm, revert persister cells, and increase susceptibility of antibiotics. However, these molecules are hydrophobic, making sustained delivery on wounded tissue a challenge. Chitosan is a natural biopolymer derived from crustacean shells that can be easily formed into injectable pastes, microbeads, particles, and electrospun nanofibers. A 72-hour test of acylated nanofiber chitosan membranes loaded with large amounts of Bupivacaine, an anesthetic shown to exhibit antimicrobial properties, found that bacterial attachment was inhibited and extended release was feasible. Future work will explore ways to use different acyl groups to control release, the use of lidocaine or other anesthetics with antimicrobial properties, the use of different bacteria to see whether common burn wound pathogens can be inhibited by these membranes, and a comb scale model to explore how the membranes can treat burn wounds.

CHAPTER SIX

Accepted Poster Abstracts

This chapter provides abstracts of the poster presentations as submitted by the author or authors to the SoSM. In consultation with the expert panel, the RAND team selected abstracts to accept for poster presentations upon evaluation of the title and the abstract. Table 6.1 provides an overview of the abstracts.

Table 6.1
Poster Presentations

Submitter	Title	Organization
Travis McQuiston	A Topical Peptide Therapeutic for Blast-Research Burn Injury	FirstString Research
Jerry Heneghan	Development of Augmented Reality Forward Surgical Care	BioMojo LLC
Chandan K. Sen	Maxillofacial Burn Trauma in Swine and Its Management	Indiana Center for Regenerative Medicine and Engineering, Indiana University School of Medicine
Laveta Stewart	Deployment-Related Burn Epidemiology: Blast & Non-Blast	Infectious Disease Clinical Research Program
George Tetz	Development of a First-in-Class Antimicrobial Agent Mul-1867	TGV-Biomed
Randall McCoy	Human Skin Regeneration for Blast-Burn Injuries	Regenicin, Inc.
Richard A. Clark	Peptide Therapy to Limit Burn and Compartment Syndrome Injury	NeoMatrix Therapeutics, Inc.
Martin J. Mangino	Designing the Next Generation Burn Resuscitation Solutions	Virginia Commonwealth University School of Medicine
Kaitlin A. Pruskowski	Fungal Infections After Blast and Thermal Injury	USAISR
M. A. Hassan Talukder	Erythropoietin in Burn-Relevant Neurogenic Muscle Atrophy	Penn State College of Medicine
Zachary Collier	A New Way of Thinking About Blast Injuries: Classification	Keck School of Medicine of the University of Southern California
John C. Elfar	Swollen Limbs and Crushed Nerves: A Role for Erythropoietin	Penn State Center for Orthopaedic Research and Translational Science
Gary S. Rogers	Portable Hypothermia Off-Loading Antimicrobial Litter	Beth Israel Lahey Health
Subhra Mandal	A Novel Combination Thermosensitive Gel Dressing for PFC	Creighton University

Table 6.1—Continued

Submitter	Title	Organization
Perenlei Enkhbaatar	Novel Approach: Autologous Keratinocyte Sheet for Burn Wound	University of Texas Medical Branch
Alison Drummond	Innovative Antimicrobial, Regenerative Blast-Injury Therapy	Cell Constructs I, LLC
Giorgio Giatsidis	Treating Blast-Related Burns with Fluorescent Light Energy	Wound Healing Research Unit, Division of Dermatology, School of Medicine, University of Pisa
Jennifer Neff	Antimicrobial Peptide Formulations for Burn Wound Protection	Allvivo Vascular
Lt Col Steven Jeffery	Kerecis (Fish Skin) for the Temporary Treatment of Burns	Royal Centre for Defence Medicine, Birmingham, United Kingdom
Aprile L. Pilon	Comparative CC10 Effects in Inhalation +/− Burn Injuries	APCBio Innovations, Inc.
David Peralta	Topical Nanoemulsion Therapy for Burn Wound Progression	BlueWillow Biologics
Kenneth A. Gruber	Symptoms of Burn Injury vs. Cachexia: Two Terms-One Syndrome	Tensive Controls
Augustine Chuang	Effective Treatment on In Vitro Blast-Burn Models	Eisenhower Army Medical Center
Nicusor Iftimia	Hand-Held Probe for Noninvasive Assessment of Burn Injuries	Physical Sciences Inc.
Elaine Christine MacAslan	Magnetic Analgesia Cuff	Cornerstone Research Group, Inc.
Lt Col Steven Jeffery	Sprayable Topical Anaesthetics for Burn-Related Injury	Royal Centre for Defence Medicine, Birmingham, United Kingdom
Jeffrey Colombe	MHS Blast Injury Prevention Standard for Dermal Burns and the Science of Burn Injury Risk to the Dermis from Explosive Blasts and Secondary Conflagrations	MITRE Corporation

Poster Presentation by Travis McQuiston

FirstString Research

A Topical Peptide Therapeutic for Blast-Research Burn Injury

Travis McQuiston, Ph.D., FirstString Research
Christina Grek, Ph.D., FirstString Research
Paul Waymack, M.D., Sc.D., FirstString Research
Gautam Ghatnekar, D.V.M., Ph.D., FirstString Research

Thermal burns are a quaternary blast injury that cause significant morbidity and mortality among U.S. combat soldiers. Thermal burn injuries account for 5–20% of military causalities and more than 60% of burned soldiers do not return to full military service because of major burn-induced disabilities. Burn conversion is a pivotal pathophysiological determinant and major obstacle in burn injury care as wound area and depth correlate to susceptibility to infection, requirement for invasive surgical procedures (e.g. excision and skin grafting), wound contracture, and excessive scarring. Currently, no U.S. Food and Drug Administration–approved (FDA-approved) therapeutic for burn injuries accelerates healing at the molecular/cellular level and prevents excessive inflammation that exacerbates burn conversion. FirstString Research has bioengineered a short peptide therapeutic, aCT1, which modulates proinflammatory connexin signaling via the stabilization of cellular junctions and the reduction of hemichannel activity. An easy-to-use, safe, topical gel formulation of aCT1 (Granexin®) has been advanced through extensive preclinical work, comprehensive investigational new drug–enabling (IND-enabling), Good Laboratory Practice–toxicology (GLP-toxicology) assessment, and multiple Phase 2 clinical trials with ongoing Phase 3 clinical trials for scar reduction and treatment of chronic wounds. Extending on the known mechanism of action of the aCT1 peptide and with support from the DoD's Medical Burn Research Program, FirstString has completed a comprehensive set of validating efficacy studies in translationally relevant animal models of acute thermal burn injury to examine the therapeutic potential of Granexin gel in mitigating burn conversion and promoting healing. In small animal models, Granexin treatment of deep partial thickness burn wounds prevents burn progression and accelerates injury reepithelialization, thus leading to a higher proportion of completely healed wounds (100% reepithelialized) in comparison to vehicle-control treatment. On Day 45, thermal burns treated with Granexin show reduced scarring and improvement in scar appearance, characterized by reduced redness, improved topography, and restoration of hair growth compared to vehicle control. In translationally relevant swine models of deep partial thickness burns, daily Granexin treatment results in improved wound healing compared to silver sulfadiazine control-treated wounds when comparing reepithelialization, collagen deposition/maturity, inflammation, and necrosis. Similarly, in full thickness thermal burn wound swine models, planimetry analyses of wounds treated post debridement with Granexin versus silver sulfadiazine showed improved healing outcomes, associated with accelerated reepithelialization as well as improved scarring outcomes at Day 56. These preclinical outcomes translate to the clinical setting as reduced necessity of skin grafting, moderated wound care regimens, and diminished chronic aesthetic and functional sequelae associated with excessive scarring. In a blast injury scenario, Granexin may be used by first responders at point of injury and during definitive care in the treatment of thermal burns. These benefits similarly apply to civilians that suffer traumatic burn injuries.

Poster Presentation by Jerry Heneghan

BioMojo, LLC

Development of Augmented Reality Forward Surgical Care

Jerry Heneghan, M.B.A., BioMojo, LLC
Brandon Conover, Ph.D., BioMojo, LLC
COL Tyler Harris, M.D., Womack Army Medical Center
Geoff Miller, M.S., Telemedicine & Advanced Technology Research Center

BioMojo, LLC in cooperation with the U.S. Army Medical Department, has developed and demonstrated an augmented reality (AR) forward surgical care system. This promises to be a crucial component of successful prolonged field care for myriad injuries on the battlefield, to include blast-related burn injuries. Our team integrated commercial-off-the-shelf (COTS) equipment with advanced software architecture to develop and demonstrate telementoring and telestration to assist medical providers in remote battlefield locations. A sample of six persons, two each of military physicians (non-surgeons), physician assistants, and special operations medics used a lightweight, rugged, wearable AR display (ODG R-7) with telestration software, bi-directional voice and video, and voice-controlled on-board magnification to receive remote guidance from surgeons across cell networks, army radios, and simulated satcom. Two procedures chosen for their complexity and surgical urgency (four-compartment fasciotomy; anterior exposure of femoral artery) were performed on synthetic-anatomy medical training manikins. The ODG R-7 preserved user peripheral vision to enable tactical situational awareness while using the device. This technology integration project demonstrated that surgical specialty is plausible in far forward environments when timely access to in-person surgical care is impossible. The operational concept was to integrate COTS items into existing telecommunication systems within the U.S. Army to create a unique operative platform. A Mastery Learning Model was developed and employed to train and assess skill performance of both the mentees (non-surgeons) and a mentor (a surgeon) during the exercise. As an integration project, the effort was not designed to reach statistical significance. Even so, the six students opened 23 of 24 fascial compartments successfully and achieved control of the proximal femoral artery on all of the six test models. The fasciotomy completion rates exceed the success rates that have been reported for attending surgeons in some studies. Blast-related burn injuries require quick response from medical personnel on the ground in order to save life and limb. Hemorrhage control and stabilization can often be achieved and maintained but only for a limited time before evacuation and surgical care are required. The deterioration of the golden hour in far forward areas necessitates prolonged field care and advanced tools to assist our warfighters. This talk will discuss the development of the AR system, the Army-approved training demonstration methodology and outcomes, lessons learned, applicability of the system to blast-related burn injuries, the roadmap for development of a fieldable system and best practices for future efforts based on our successful demonstration.

Disclaimer: The views expressed herein are those of the author(s) and do not reflect the official policy or position of the U.S. government or any branch therein.

Poster Presentation by Chandan K. Sen

Indiana Center for Regenerative Medicine and Engineering, Indiana University School of Medicine

Maxillofacial Burn Trauma in Swine and Its Management
Sashwati Roy, Ph.D., Indiana Center for Regenerative Medicine and Engineering, Indiana University School of Medicine
Nandini Ghosh, Ph.D., Indiana Center for Regenerative Medicine and Engineering, Indiana University School of Medicine
Amitava Das, Ph.D., Indiana Center for Regenerative Medicine and Engineering, Indiana University School of Medicine
Vinoj Gopalakrishnan, Ph.D., Indiana Center for Regenerative Medicine and Engineering, Indiana University School of Medicine

Chandan K. Sen, Ph.D., Indiana Center for Regenerative Medicine and Engineering, Indiana University School of Medicine

Background. The heat of an explosive blast causes flash burns of the face not protected by armor. These burns involve the skin, underlying muscle and often even the bone. Because of the high heat involved, fourth degree burns are common. Maxillofacial thermal injuries cause major facial disfiguration that burdens the subject socially, emotionally, psychologically and functionally such as oral incompetence. Critical and unique facial characteristics in thermal injury of the face include ectropion (epithelial-ocular junction), eversion of the lip (epithelial-oral junction), skin contracture and scar formation. Compared to scar response in other parts of the body, facial scar contractures are much more severe. The objective of this DoD sponsored current work was to establish the first pre-clinical experimental model to study burn-induced scarring of the face and to test the healing outcomes in response to a glycerin-based wound dressing Elasto-Gel in porcine model.

Methods. Roughly 50% facial surface of the white pig was subjected fourth degree burn involving the bone. Wounds were treated with placebo (Acticoat) or Elasto-Gel (SouthWest Tech) dressings that were changed once a week for 84 days. Progression of burn wound healing was followed using non-invasive imaging: (a) laser speckle microperfusion imaging (LSI); (b) harmonic ultrasound imaging with Doppler (HUSD) for tissue stiffness and blood supply; and (c) computed tomography (CT) with angiography for 3D reconstruction of the facial tissues and their vasculature. Additionally, wound inflammation, angiogenesis and remodeling were examined using standard immunohistochemistry.

Results. CT and ultrasound imaging established fourth degree burn with bone involvement showing severe deficits including ectropion, oral eversion and contracture, excessive scarring as well as drooling during eating. All of these characteristics are consistent with manifestations commonly noted in humans with facial burn. Intense contracture and scarring were evident at d84 post-burn. Vascular and bone deficits ($n = 7$) were visualized using LSI, HUSD and CT imaging. The specific areas of the face involving mucocutaneous junctions as opposed to scar healed in a different manner. The abundance of macrophages was significantly lower.

Conclusion. This maiden pre-clinical model recapitulates features characteristic of human facial burns involving the mucocutaneous junctions. Histopathological analysis revealed differential inflammatory, vascularization and scarring responses at anatomic locations. This work constitutes maiden report on a porcine model of severe facial burn contracture. Application of Elasto-Gel dressing improved facial scar outcomes.

Disclaimer: The study was supported by USMRAA # W81XWH-16-P-0259.

Poster Presentation by Laveta Stewart

Infectious Disease Clinical Research Program

Deployment-Related Burn Epidemiology: Blast & Non-Blast
Laveta Stewart, MSc, M.D., Ph.D., Infectious Disease Clinical Research Program
Faraz Shaikh, M.S., Infectious Disease Clinical Research Program
Dana Blyth, M.D., Brooke Army Medical Center
Wesley Campbell, M.D., Walter Reed National Military Medical Center
David Tribble, M.D., DrPH, Infectious Disease Clinical Research Program

Background: Combat-related burn injuries represent 5% of casualties evacuated from operations in Iraq and Afghanistan (2003–2005). The majority of burns sustained during combat are due to blasts (e.g. improvised explosive devices). Burn-related infections, specifically bloodstream infections (BSIs), are an important cause of mortality. *Pseudomonas aeruginosa, Klebsiella pneumoniae, Acinetobacter calcoaceticus-baumannii* (ACB) complex, and *Staphylococcus aureus* are frequently isolated from burn wounds. We assessed the epidemiology of deployment-related burn injuries (blast and non-blast) and their outcomes among the Trauma Infectious Disease Outcomes Study population (2009–2014).

Methods: Wounded personnel were included in the analysis if they sustained ≥ 1 burn injury (2009–2014), were admitted to Landstuhl Regional Medical Center (LRMC), and were transferred to a participating U.S. military hospital. Injury characteristics, microbiology, and clinical outcomes were assessed. Infections attributable to burns were defined as superficial soft tissue infections (SSTIs) and osteomyelitis at the site of the burn, as well as BSI, pneumonia, and sepsis. Subjects were further evaluated and compared by blast and non-blast mechanisms of injury.

Results: Among 2699 combat casualties transferred to a participating U.S. military hospital, 276 (10%) sustained at least one burn-related injury; 206 (75%) were classified as blast-injured, and 70 (25%) were injured via non-blast mechanisms (e.g., electrical burn and fire). Burn subjects were primarily male (98.6%) and injured in Afghanistan (84.4%) with Total Body Surface Area (TBSA) > 20% reported for 19%. Compared to non-blast burn patients, blast-injured burn patients were more severely injured (median injury severity score: 17.5 vs 4; $p = 0.001$) and had a higher first documented shock index (median: 0.73 vs 0.66; $p = 0.008$). Blast-injured burn patients also had a longer U.S. hospital length of stay (median days: 19.5 vs 7; $p = 0.001$), were more frequently admitted to the ICU in the U.S. (47% vs 24%; $p = 0.001$), and required mechanical ventilation in the U.S. (22% vs 16%; $p = 0.001$). Colonization with multidrug-resistant organisms at LRMC admission was more common in blast-injured burn patients compared to non-blast burn patients (11% vs 1.4%; $p = 0.001$). While % TBSA was not significantly different, blast-injured patients had a higher proportion of burns on the head, face, neck (62% vs 46%; $p = 0.016$) or shoulder (10% vs 0%; $p = 0.005$) vs non-blast burn patients who were more frequently burned on the hands, digits, and lower extremity. Non-blast burn patients had more partial (77% vs 52%) and full-thickness burns (38% vs 32%) compared to blast-injured patients ($p = 0.001$). Overall, BSIs and pneumonia were diagnosed in 11% and 13% of burn patients, respectively. Predominant organisms isolated from burn wounds, blood, or respiratory specimens were ACB complex and *P. aeruginosa*. Coagulase-negative *Staphylococcus* was the most frequent among blood specimens and *S. aureus, Streptococcus spp.*, and *Escherichia coli* were largely isolated from respiratory specimens.

Conclusions: Blast-related trauma is often accompanied by burn injuries; however, short- and long-term outcomes associated with these injuries are not well understood. Despite higher injury severity and polytrauma among blast-injured burn patients, burn-specific severity measures did not differ by blast status. Burn site location differences by blast and non-blast mechanisms emphasize a review of personal protective equipment.

Disclaimer(s): The views expressed are those of the authors and do not reflect the official views of the Uniformed Services University of the Health Sciences.

Poster Presentation by George Tetz

TGV-Biomed

Development of a First-in-Class Antimicrobial Agent Mul-1867

George Tetz, M.D., Ph.D., TGV-Biomed
Victor Tetz, M.D., Ph.D., Human Microbiology Institute
Yakov Kogan, Ph.D., M.B.A., TGV-Biomed

Background: Bacterial and fungal infections are a major problem both to the military (combat) field and blast-related burn injuries in particular. Challenges include mixed biofilms, formed by different microorganisms, including bacterial-fungal mix. Particularly resistant are biofilms formed by spore forming bacteria, predominantly of *Bacillus spp.* and *Clostridium spp.*, which are extremely poorly treated due to the resistance of spores to antimicrobial agents. Commonly used antibiotics and sanitizers are ineffective against microbial biofilms and spore forming bacteria. Mul-1867 is a first-in-class within the guanidine group of surface acting drug candidates with a unique nanostructure that allows significantly improved treatment of biofilm-associated wound infections, including those formed by spore forming and multi-resistant microorganisms.

Methods: The minimum inhibitory concentration (MIC) against various aerobic and anaerobic Gram-positive and Gram-negative bacterial and fungal isolates was determined and compared to antibiotics and antiseptics currently used (including military) according to Clinical and Laboratory Standards Institute (CLSI) criteria. A "Time-kill" antibiofilm study was performed to ensure that Mul-1867 can act within less than 10 min against biofilms formed by skin and wound clinical isolates (48-h-old) of Gram-positive, Gram-negative bacteria and fungi. Data were reported as the Minimum biofilm eliminating concentration (MBEC). Bacterial strains: *Bacillus spp* (N20), *Enterococcus spp* (N20), *E. coli* (N10), *Klebsiella spp* (N20), *Pseudomonas aeruginosa* (N40), *Staphylococcus spp* (including MRSA/VRSA) (N40), *Streptococcus epidermidis* (N30), *Proteus spp* (N20), *Citrobacter spp* (N20), *Acinetobacter spp* (N20), fungi associated with wound and blast-related burn infections, including *Candida spp* (N15) and *Aspergillus spp* (N15). Cell cytotoxicity of Mul-1867 was tested by the modified MTT assay.

Results: Mul-1867 was shown to be effective against a variety of bacteria including multi-resistant strains. It exhibited significant activity against all isolates of Gram-positive and Gram-negative bacteria that were resistant to amikacin, aztreonam, ceftazidime, meropenem, piperacillin, tobramycin, alcohols and chlorhexidine, as well as against susceptible and control strains. Mul-1867 inhibited the growth of all the gram-positive microorganisms tested, with MIC values ranging from 0.03 to 0.5 mg/L and all gram-negative bacteria with MIC from 0.25–8 mg/L. In all cases MIC values of Mul-1867 against bacteria were considerably (from 32 to 512 times) lower than those of antibiotics and sanitizers used as the positive controls. There was no statistically significant difference between the activity of Mul-1867 against the susceptible vs. antibiotic resistant strains. Mul-1867 was effective against 48-hr-old bacterial and fungal biofilms within contact times of 15–60 sec, showing more from 32 to over 1000X more effectivity as compared with antibiotics and sanitizers. Mul-1867 was the only antimicrobial tested being able to eliminate and prevent recurrence of biofilms of spore forming bacteria. The compound did not exhibit any statistically significant cytotoxicity against MDCK cells, as tested by the MTT assay 4 h after challenging with Mul-1867.

Conclusions: Mul-1867 is a novel antimicrobial active against a wide range of multi-resistant organisms (Gram-positive and Gram-negative bacteria and fungi) at safe concentrations for humans. Overall, these data indicate that Mul-1867 is a promising antimicrobial drug candidate for the treatment and mitigating the impact of biofilm-challenged blast-related burn injuries.

Poster Presentation by Randall McCoy

Regenicin, Inc.

Human Skin Regeneration for Blast-Burn Injuries

Randall McCoy, B.S., Regenicin, Inc.
Scott A. Blow, B.S., M.B.A., Regenicin, Inc.

NovaDerm® can save lives and restore dignity and quality of life to military blast-burn victims. NovaDerm is the only autologous cultured skin substitute for full thickness burns that is grown from the patient's own cells. In just 28 days or less, enough skin is grown to cover the entire body with only two grafting procedures. In addition, NovaDerm has a shelf life of 2 weeks, thus enabling the physician to choose grafting times optimal for the patient.

Utilizing a small harvested section of the patient's own skin, new skin can be grown up to four hundred times the harvested section's original size. This living self-to-self skin-graft-tissue forms permanent skin that will grow with the patient and not be rejected by the immune system, a critical problem with the porcine and cadaver skin grafts used today.

Without the skin (the largest human organ) covering the body, a person would quickly expire. The faster a patient is fully covered with skin, the higher the probability of survival. Traditional burn treatment protocol is lengthy, extraordinarily painful and very expensive. NovaDerm greatly benefits severe burn patients in all three of these areas.

NovaDerm's benefits would be extraordinary for military blast-burn patients:

- Minimize time to full wound closure to limit infection
- Minimize number of initial surgeries (from as many as 8–12 to only 2)
- Minimize painful rounds of donor skin harvesting for grafting (substantially reduce or eliminate harvesting)
- Minimize time to discharge (reduce from as long as multiple years to several months)
- Minimize need for subsequent revision surgeries
- Minimize total cost to treat patient (by 50% or more)
- Eliminate need for immunosuppressants (skin is genetic matching and thus no rejection).

NovaDerm can make it possible for a major burn victim to return to normal daily function in six months or less, versus as long as several years under traditional treatment protocol. In addition, current major burn treatment methodology can require from 90 to 365 hospital stay days. NovaDerm treatment can reduce hospital day stays to fewer than 50 days. NovaDerm skin is the patient's own skin. It moves, grows and wears just like the real thing because it is the patient's own skin.

In effort to return (as much as is humanly possible) some normalcy and restore quality of life to the highest extent possible, NovaDerm can serve a significant role in improving the lives of our military sisters and brothers who are injured due to blast burns.

Disclaimer: Approaching final phase of FDA trials.

Poster Presentation by Richard A. Clark

NeoMatrix Therapeutics, Inc.

Peptide Therapy to Limit Burn and Compartment Syndrome Injury

Richard A. Clark, M.D., NeoMatrix Therapeutics, Inc.
Fubao Lin, Ph.D., NeoMatrix Therapeutics, Inc.

Burns and compartment syndrome (CS) in underlying muscles are major problems after blast injury. NeoMatrix Therapeutics, Inc. (NMT) has developed multi-functional peptide-based, scalable therapies for burns: cP12 (designated Orphan Drug and Fast Track) and cNP8 (67% homologous to cP12). An optimal dose (0.01 mg/kg) of cP12, as a single 30-min intravenous (iv) infusion, initiated 2–4 h post-burn, limits burn conversion and speeds healing in pigs at 14 d post-burn as judged by % wounds completely healed (70% vs 30% control). From these efficacy studies, coupled with preclinical safety studies, NMT launched a Phase 1 Clinical Trial (CT), July, 2019 (W81XWH-18-2-0059). The clinical trial should be successfully completed by early 2020. NMT also engineered a cP12-related peptide, cNP8, to be elastase-resistant. The cNP8 peptide gives a healing response similar to cP12 in burns and significantly reduces scarring at 0.01 mg/kg with a 30-min iv infusion, initiated 12–24 h post-burn (Lin et al., 2020). cNP8 has completed preclinical efficacy and safety studies (W81XWH-15-C-0043). Remaining IND-enabling studies will commence pending Combat Readiness program support. From dog safety studies, we found that cNP8 at 20x optimal dose can be delivered as a 1-min bolus iv injection, rather than a 30-min iv infusion, the currently approved iv protocol (active cP12 IND). Importantly, preclinical studies of cP12 and cNP8 efficacy in CS have been recently proposed (Armed Forces Institute of Regenerative Medicine [AFIRM III] pending). We believe these therapies will work synergistically (Burn Program Idea Award pending), but can be used separately. Such scalable iv therapies for blast injury would be greatly beneficial under hazards of Prolonged Field Care (PFC).

Mechanistically, the root cause of burn conversion and CS is microvascular ischemia. From porcine burn studies, red blood cell (RBC) aggregates, not microthrombi, occlude peri-burn microvasculature. cP12, given at optimal dose and time to increase healing and decrease scarring, markedly reduces RBC occlusion (Asif et al., 2016), most likely by microvascular dilation (Frame et al., 2017). In addition, cP12 (Lin et al., 2014) and cNP8 (Lin et al., 2020) increase survival and growth of skin and muscle cells under nutrient deprivation, reactive oxygen species (ROS) generation, or endoplasmic reticulum (ER) stress. Together these mechanistic attributes of cP12 and cNP8 help elucidate why the peptides have such robust ability to speed healing and reduce scarring in burns and likely in CS.

Poster Presentation by Martin J. Mangino

Virginia Commonwealth University School of Medicine

Designing the Next Generation Burn Resuscitation Solutions

Martin J. Mangimo, Ph.D., Virginia Commonwealth University School of Medicine
Michael Feldman, M.D., Virginia Commonwealth University School of Medicine

Three million patients in the U.S. are hospitalized with burns and over 240,000 die from these injuries each year. In severe burns, fluid loss and cardiovascular collapse are the main life-threatening problems. Intravascular fluid loss occurs from direct capillary leak in injured capillaries and from intracellular water accumulation following mitochondrial failure from thermal injury. Loss of ATP-dependent cell volume control mechanisms results in tissue swelling and microvascular compression that further aggravates capillary flow at resuscitation leading to more ischemia in a self-amplifying cycle. Using the Parkland Protocol, as much as 15–20 liters of IV crystalloids may be administered to severely burned patients within the first 24 hours. However, massive delivery of sodium and water exacerbates these problems by promoting more sodium and water entry into cells, which are already compromised by depressed Na/K ATPase driven pumps. To break this cycle, we have developed novel IV crystalloid resuscitation solutions containing customized hydrophilic polyethylene glycol (PEG) polymers that rapidly and non-energetically transfer water and sodium out of the cells and into the capillaries. This serves to both decompress the capillaries to reduce resistance to flow and to reload the capillaries with isotonic volume to restore driving pressures for flow. Together, both promote robust capillary flow and efficient exchange of oxygen to tissues to support normal function and burn repair. These polymers also may serve to rebuild the endothelial glycocalyx in tissues damaged by burns and reduce secondary cellular inflammation. In lethal models of hypovolemia causing similar shock as seen in burn shock, PEG based IV resuscitation solutions are highly effective at reducing local tissue water accumulation, restoring central hemodynamics, improving capillary flow and oxygen transfer, and dramatically promoting survival from lethal injury using extremely low volumes of IV resuscitation compared to the Parkland protocol. Furthermore, the solutions are stable under harsh environmental conditions where they can support far forward field use in badly burned patients awaiting long transport times. The paradigm of burn resuscitation has changed where central hemodynamic and vascular volume outcomes are replaced by approaches that restore capillary oxygen exchange by non-energetically restoring cell, tissue, and capillary volumes that drive convective capillary exchange.

Poster Presentation by Kaitlin A. Pruskowski

USAISR

Fungal Infections After Blast and Thermal Injury

Kaitlin A. Pruskowski, Pharm.D., USAISR
Julie A. Rizzo, M.D., USAISR
Leopoldo C. Cancio, M.D., USAISR

Background: Invasive fungal wound infections have been reported after combat-related blast injuries sustained in Operations Iraqi Freedom and Enduring Freedom. Systemic antifungal agents are commonly used as an adjunct to urgent surgical debridement. There is currently controversy in defining the depth of fungal invasion, which is the most critical factor that determines the treatment strategy. The objective of this study was to describe fungal infections in blast injury patients admitted to our burn center.

Methods: This was a retrospective chart review. Subjects who were admitted between January 2004 and February 2019, received a systemic antifungal agent, and experienced a blast injury were included. Culture and histopathology results were recorded.

Results: Eighty-one patients were included. Seventy-five subjects (92.6%) were active-duty service members at the time of injury. Seventy-nine (97.5%) subjects were male, with an average age of 27.4 ± 7.8 years. The average burn size was 51.4 ± 25.3% TBSA. Twenty-seven subjects (33.3%) died during their hospital stay. The 75 subjects had 157 cultures positive for fungi, including 130 tissue cultures. The most common genera isolated were *Aspergillus* (*n* = 148), followed by *Candida* (*n* = 106), *Fusarium* (*n* = 16), and *Mucor* (*n* = 12). Four subjects (57.1%) who grew *Mucor* died, as compared to 13 (52%) who grew *Aspergillus*, 5 (50%) who grew *Fusarium*, and 10 (32.3%) who grew *Candida*. Subjects who grew multiple genera of fungi had a higher mortality rate (52.9%), as compared to subjects who grew a single genus (34.4%) or did not have fungal culture growth (21.9%). For histopathology, 33 (40.7%) had results that showed fungus in non-viable tissue; the average time to fungus in non-viable tissue was 19.1 ± 18.2 days. Twenty-one subjects (25.9%) had results that showed fungus in viable tissue; the average time to fungus in viable tissue was 22.5 ± 20.3 days. Fourteen subjects (17.3%) had results that showed angioinvasion; the average time to angioinvasion was 24.2 ± 22.3 days from injury. Subjects who had fungus in viable tissue had the highest mortality rate (71.4%), followed by angioinvasion (64.3%), and fungus in non-viable tissue (33.3%). The 75 subjects received 121 courses of systemic antifungals. The average duration of therapy was 12.3 ± 13.6 days. The most common antifungals ordered were voriconazole (*n* = 58), fluconazole (*n* = 53), and liposomal amphotericin B (*n* = 42).

Conclusion: Invasive fungal infection after blast injury had a high mortality rate of 33.3%. Early recognition and management of fungal infections is paramount to patient survival. A consensus is needed on how to best define the depth and level of invasion of fungal wound infections, and to determine the optimal treatment duration of systemic antifungal agents for these patients.

Disclaimer(s): The views expressed in this abstract are those of the authors and do not reflect the official policy or position of the U.S. Army, DoD, or U.S. Government.

Poster Presentation by M. A. Hassan Talukder

Penn State College of Medicine

Erythropoietin in Burn-Relevant Neurogenic Muscle Atrophy

M. A. Hassan Talukder, M.D., Ph.D., Penn State College of Medicine
Jung Il Lee, M.D., Penn State College of Medicine
Mary O'Brien, B.S., Penn State College of Medicine

Zara Karuman, M.S., Penn State College of Medicine
John Elfar, M.D., Penn State College of Medicine

Background: Severe burns in the limb are known to cause irrecoverable injury to nerves. Burn-induced local ischemia and edema can lead to compartment syndrome followed by nerve compression and muscle ischemia. Almost all severe burn victims are also anemic from blood loss and hemolysis in the hyper-inflammatory state of burn injury. Erythropoietin (EPO) is a pleiotropic hormone with potent erythropoietic, cytoprotective, angiogenic, and anti-inflammatory properties. We reasoned that post-burn nerve compression–induced neurogenic muscle atrophy will benefit from EPO treatment. Both EPO and EPO receptors (EPOR) are present in muscle and peripheral nerve. This study was designed to explore the beneficial effect of EPO and EPOR on neurogenic muscle atrophy and functional recovery following burn-injury-relevant nerve compression injury.

Methods: Schwann cell–specific EPOR knockout (MPZ-Cre EPOR f/f) and wild-type (WT) mice were assigned to moderate sciatic nerve crush injury and followed for 3, 7 and 14 days with one dose of immediate post-injury EPO (5000 units/kg, intraperitoneal) or saline treatment. Post-injury muscle atrophy and functional recovery were evaluated.

Results: Neurogenic muscle atrophy was comparable (~12%, $n = 7$) between saline-treated WT and EPOR-knockout mice. EPO treatment abolished muscle atrophy in WT mice (< 4%, $n = 7$), whereas muscle atrophy was exacerbated in EPO-treated EPOR knockout mice (19%, $P < 0.001$, $n = 7$) and it was significantly different from EPO-treated WT mice ($P < 0.001$). Post-injury limb function was comparable between WT and EPOR knockout mice in the saline group. While EPO treatment markedly accelerated post-injury function in WT mice, functional recovery in EPOR knockout mice remained significantly impaired.

Conclusion: These findings provide direct evidence that EPO via EPOR prevents muscle atrophy and improves post-injury functional recovery following nerve crush injury and open a new window for game changing therapeutic opportunity of EPO in blast-related burn-injury-induced neurogenic muscle loss, rehabilitation and readiness.

Poster Presentation by Zachary Collier

Keck School of Medicine of the University of Southern California

A New Way of Thinking About Blast Injuries: Classification

Zachary Collier, M.D., Keck School of Medicine of the University of Southern California
K. J. Choi, B.A., Keck School of Medicine of the University of Southern California
I. F. Hulsebos, B.S., Keck School of Medicine of the University of Southern California
C. H. Pham, M.D., Keck School of Medicine of the University of Southern California
T. J. Gillenwater, M.D., Keck School of Medicine of the University of Southern California

Introduction: Blast injuries present unique challenges to civilian and military healthcare providers because of the complex and often severe nature of injuries spanning numerous anatomical regions and systems. The combination of direct shockwave, re-pressurization phenomenon, thermal and chemical components, and high velocity projectiles results in significantly variable depths and distributions of injury that are frequently contaminated with bacteria-containing foreign debris. Due to these factors, we devised a novel wound-focused classification system for implementation during triage and management of blast injuries to optimize outcomes.

Methods: A retrospective analysis of patients treated by our ABA-certified burn center for blast-related injuries from September 1, 2014, to October 31, 2019, was performed. Demographics, mechanism and distribution of injuries, interventions, and outcomes were evaluated. Injuries were classified using a wound-focused classification composed of four zones. Zone 1 included areas closest to the blast epicenter that had total or near-total tissue loss from the blast. Zone 2 comprised adjacent areas with thermal and chemical burns. Zone 3 involved any distant site outside of Zones 1 and 2 where shrapnel created additional wounds. Zone 4 included injuries arising from barotrauma.

Results: We identified 64 patients who were mostly male (84%), averaging 38 years of age. Mechanisms of injury included fireworks (19%), industrial accidents (16%), volatile fuels and drug labs (46%), and others including can, battery, and lighter explosions (19%). All mechanisms had equivalent frequency of Zone 2 injuries with an average TBSA of 17 ± 17%. Volatile fuels caused the highest TBSA (21.9%), and industrial accidents caused the most full thickness burns (30% vs average 23%). Fireworks had five-fold (17% vs. 3%) more Zone 3 and three-fold (25% vs 8%) more Zone 4 injuries compared to the other mechanisms. Two-thirds (4 out of 6) of patients presenting to our burn team over 24 hours after initial injury had infections—a four-fold increase compared to non-delayed presentations (66.7% vs. 13.8%). Overall, 45% required surgery (31% grafting, 7% flaps) with 9.4% having concomitant injuries and 2% requiring fracture repair. Some patients (42%) required ICU admission or intubation although the industrial accident group had the highest rate (60%).

Conclusion: Overall, civilians with blast injuries most often required admission for management of the Zone 2 component. Interestingly, different blast mechanisms resulted in distinct patterns of injury although fireworks had the greatest number of Zone 1, 3, and 4 injuries with an equivalent incidence of Zone 2 across the mechanisms. When patients were thoroughly assessed and treated according to the zone classification, less complications occurred and overall outcomes were improved. Application of this classification system to military blast injuries may help identify unique, predictable zonal distribution patterns for specific ordinance or blast types that would facilitate early zone directed interventions to optimize resuscitative and reconstructive efforts.

Poster Presentation by John C. Elfar

Penn State Center for Orthopaedic Research and Translational Science

Swollen Limbs and Crushed Nerves: A Role for Erythropoietin

Prem Kumar Govindappa, D.V.M., Ph.D., Penn State Center for Orthopaedic Research and Translational Science
M. A. Hassan Talukder, M.B.B.S., Ph.D., Penn State Center for Orthopaedic Research and Translational Science
Anagha Gurjar, Ph.D., Penn State Center for Orthopaedic Research and Translational Science
John Hegarty, M.S., Penn State Center for Orthopaedic Research and Translational Science
John C. Elfar, M.D., F.A.C.S., Penn State Center for Orthopaedic Research and Translational Science

Background: Post burn resuscitation commonly involves limb fascial and skin decompression via escharotomy to protect against swelling-induced tissue loss and compressive nerve injury. Post-burn compressive nerve injury is common and burns themselves can result in crushing of the nerve by local tissue swelling. Erythropoietin (EPO) is a pleiotropic hormone with potent tissue-protective properties in preclinical models of traumatic, ischemic, and inflammatory injuries. We found that EPO is protective in the setting of nerve compression and crush injuries independent of burns, where EPO treatment is indicated for other reasons (anemia, hemolysis, etc.). Critical to understanding EPO's role is knowing how severe injury itself can alter efficacy.

This study was designed to investigate the neuroprotective effect of EPO with a new regimen in burn-injury-relevant severe nerve crush injury.

Methods: Mice were assigned to sham, severe crush injury alone (saline) and severe crush injury with EPO groups. Sciatic nerve crush injury was performed using calibrated forceps for 30 sec, and EPO (5000 IU/kg) or sterile saline (0.1 mL) was administered intraperitoneally immediately post injury and daily for 2 days afterward. Functional recovery was assessed on post-injury day 1, 3, 7, 14 and 21 by sciatic function index (SFI), von Frey testing, and grip strength evaluation. Nerves were also subjected to gene and protein expression analysis.

Results: Compared to saline, EPO treatment significantly improved post-injury motor function (SFI), grip strength, and sensory function. Functional improvement was associated with a markedly better mRNA expression profile of inflammatory, anti-inflammatory, angiogenesis, and myelination related genes in the injured nerves. EPO also preserved the protein expression of neurofilament, myelin, and capillaries in the injured nerves.

Conclusions: We demonstrate an effective EPO dose regimen directly translatable to the severely injured limb where nerve injury often co-exists with other indications for EPO use. The 3-day EPO treatment regimen augments functional recovery by mitigating inflammatory, anti-inflammatory, angiogenesis, and myelination components of nerve injury. These findings suggest that EPO might offer a therapeutic opportunity to transform blast-related burn-injury-induced severe nerve injury.

Poster Presentation by Gary S. Rogers

Beth Israel Lahey Health

Portable Hypothermia Off-Loading Antimicrobial Litter

Gary S. Rogers, M.D., Beth Israel Lahey Health
Alexander White, B.S., University of North Carolina School of Medicine
Steven E. Wolf, M.D., University of Texas Medical Branch

Both combat-related as well as civilian burn/blast trauma are associated with significant patient mortality. Pathogen-laden high-velocity blast particles can embed in skin and soft tissues producing deep-seated infections. Rapid blood loss, loss of skin barrier due to burn trauma and inability to generate and maintain adequate body temperature can quickly progress to hypothermic shock. Prolonged periods of field care and extended transport time on rigid litters can escalate the occurrence of pressure ulcers. Addressing these 3 complications of combat-related trauma is critical when designing new methods of casualty medical transport.

Rogers Sciences, Inc. (RSI) has developed an opto-electronic solution to manage wounds in a safe and sustainable manner that does not incorporate the use of drugs or chemicals. The phototherapeutic approach harnesses light in the visible blue spectrum, avoiding harmful ultraviolet wavelengths, to effectively decontaminate wounds. The antimicrobial properties of the device have demonstrated > 5 log kill of the 6 major gram positive and negative bacteria that cause skin wound infections including methicillin-resistant *Staph. Aureus* and Vancomycin-resistant *enterococcus*. The device also demonstrated a 5.8-log reduction of *Acinetobacter* and significant reduction of *Candida* and *Aspergillus* species that were subjected to the therapy in-vitro. The device can be placed directly onto the wound and remain in place for up to 7 days. IRB approved pilot clinical studies have demonstrated the antimicrobial effects and lack of tissue toxicity. This approach has the potential to prevent the onset of infection in burn and blast wounds during evacuation from battlefield to trauma center and transport from trauma center to tertiary care facility. Preventing infection and the onset of biofilm formation in acute wounds will reduce morbidity of wound complications as well as reduce medical supply-chain needs and cost of care.

RSI's patented Lumina24 BLU technology, fabricated as a burn-blanket, is being modified into a combat transport pad that incorporates infrared illumination to prevent hypothermia. Unlike Mylar trauma blankets or Reddy-Heat (Techtrade, LLC) that can take > 20 minutes to reach operating temperature, RSI's transport pad will reach 37C within 100 seconds of application. This should significantly reduce morbidity, particularly the onset of coagulopathies in both military and civilian trauma settings. The small foot-print and lightweight (under 8 lbs.) of the technology will facilitate storage in dismounted, ground vehicle, shipboard, and air platform evacuation litter settings The illumination technology is being tested with a novel alternating air bladder system, field deployable, to prevent the onset of pressure ulcers. The benefits of the Portable Hypothermia Off-loading Antimicrobial Litter (PHOAL) under development span acute trauma management to prolonged field care. By taking preventive measures that focus on dynamic off-loading, antiseptic phototherapy, and stable thermal management, medical military personnel are ensuring that combat casualty patients have the highest chances of survival. The PHOAL trauma transport system will be a rapidly deployable advanced burn/blast wound intervention that will provide antimicrobial and anti-biofilm phototherapy, off-loading and hypothermia prevention. This will result in better long-term outcomes, decreasing mortality, morbidity, burn unit length of stay and resource utilization.

Disclaimer: Rogers Sciences Inc. is a start-up Medical Device company initially funded via the NIH Small Business Innovation Research (SBIR) mechanism.

Poster Presentation by Subhra Mandal

Creighton University

A Novel Combination Thermosensitive Gel Dressing for PFC
Subhra Mandal, Ph.D., Creighton University

Pavan Kumar Parthipati, Ph.D., Creighton University
Christopher J. Destache, Pharm.D., Creighton University

Background: During a conflict, burn injuries significantly contribute to soldier morbidity and mortality. Globally, burns account for 5–20% casualties of all injuries. In the future conflict, potential increases in burn casualties are expected. The major cause will be the distance from battlefield medical care facilities and delays in transportation to a burn care center. Therefore, potential strategic on-site burn care intervention in a pre-hospital setting is needed to support "prolonged field care (PFC)" that withstands delays. The overall objective of this research strategy is to formulate novel ideal multi-component-loaded combination thermo-sensitive (cTMS) gel dressing that provides everything that is necessary to improve overall healing time, reduce infection risk, promote absorption of wound fluids and exudates, and provide mechanical strength to accelerate healing. This cTMS gel dressing is applicable to all acute burn wound types to support PFC. The long-term goal of our strategy is to formulate an advanced dressing material that creates an environment as close as possible to the ideal. The goal is to promote pain relief, infection protection, and healing during PFC, in a form that enables non-medical or medical first responders to provide appropriate burn care, to ensure better long-term outcomes.

Method: We have fabricated a reproducible, stable and scalable TMS gel with the critical gelation temperature (Tc) $\geq$ 28°C at different pH conditions. Further, in the cTMS gel, LA nano-formulations loaded with antibiotics were incorporated. The LA antibiotic NPs in the cTMS gel was evaluated for sustained release potency. In the next aim, we evaluate and select out the most effective cTMS gel formulation that is non-cytotoxic; permits molecular exchange; cell migration, growth, and differentiation.

Results and Discussion: The fabricated cTMS gel demonstrated a critical gelation temperature (Tc) of 27 ± 2°C, ($n = 4$ batches) at different pH conditions and serosanguineous fluid absorption does not infer with their thermogelation properties. Our study demonstrates TMS gel fluid absorbance is a gradual process due to gel capillary action (t1/2 9 h) and > 60% of liquid was adsorbed within 24 h. Further, antibiotics release kinetics studies illustrate that the LA antibiotic NPs cTMS gel (pH 4.5) induces 75% and 40% antibiotic release respectively from poly lactic-co-glycolic acid (PLGA) NP and CAP NP to support instant first-line defense and promote healing at the time of application to support PFC. This study also reflected that the TMS gel matrix doesn't hinder transport and therefore material exchange rate is very fast, (i.e. within ~3 h of incubation 50% of the drug gets distributed from TMS gel to the 1X phosphate-buffered saline (PBS) solution.

Conclusion & future directions: The proposed multi-component-loaded dressing cTMS gel will provide all components needed to improve overall healing time, reduce infection, promote wound fluid absorption, and provide mechanical strength to accelerate healing irrespective of the type of wound and is applicable to all acute burn wound types. Our future aim is to design the cTMS gel with LA combination nano/macro formulations loaded with antibiotics, analgesic, growth factors; and to verify healing efficacy of optimized LA combination nano/macro formulations cTMS gel on a porcine model.

Poster Presentation by Perenlei Enkhbaatar

University of Texas Medical Branch

Novel Approach: Autologous Keratinocyte Sheet for Burn Wound

Perenlei Enkhbaatar, M.D., Ph.D., University of Texas Medical Branch

Introduction: Burn injuries are an increasing concern among military Service members. Timely coverage of a burn wound is critical for improving survival and long-term life quality. However, lack or limited availability of autologous donor skin complicates treatment of large burns. Use of cultured autologous keratinocyte sheets (aKSs) has been proposed; however, this approach has not been translated to clinical practice due to complications. We hypothesize that enzyme (Dispase) used for aKSs detachment from dish compromises the extracellular matrix (ECM) and negatively impacts cell quality. We aimed to test efficacy of non-enzymatically detached aKSs, using novel technology.

Methods: Primary ovine keratinocytes were cultured in novel temperature-responsive dish and were detached by temperature reduction without using enzyme (T sheets). Cells were also cultured in conventional dish to be detached by Dispase (D sheets). First, in vitro studies investigated integrity of sheets and characterized ECM. Second, efficacy of these sheets was compared in vivo. Six full thickness skin burns (5 x 5 cm) were induced in sheep dorsum under anesthesia and analgesia. To mimic clinical scenario, burned skin was excised at 24 h and grafted with ovine cadaver skin. At 3 weeks, rejected cadaver skin epidermis was debrided, and wounds were covered with T or D sheets and monitored for 2 weeks (macro and microscopic methods).

Results: (1) In vitro: Cultured keratinocytes in both dishes formed firm multilayer sheets within 3 weeks, mimicking time of cadaver skin rejection. Sheet thickness was significantly higher in T sheets (18.1 ± 0.9 um) vs. D sheets (11.6 ± 1.2) with preserved ECM and cytoskeleton proteins. D sheet size was reduced by ~30% after detachment, whereas T sheets were intact. Following share stress, fragmentation and number of disassociated cells were significantly higher in D sheets.

(2) In vivo: Epithelialization percentage was significantly higher in T sheets: 59.1 ± 5.7% and 95.1 ± 1.3% at day 7 and 81.1 ± 6.0% and 98.5 ± 1.3% at day 14 in D and T sheet wounds, respectively. Dermal-epidermal junction was well defined in T sheet wounds (continuous lamina densa and higher hemi-desmosomes) with less hemorrhage, ulceration and neutrophils.

Conclusion: Effects of non-enzymatically detached aKSs with preserved ECM on burn wound healing are superior to those of Dispase-detached sheets. Our study builds a strong platform for potential clinical trials to test efficacy of T sheets in burn patients.

Disclaimer: Staff members of Translational Intensive Care Unit at the University of Texas Medical Branch Galveston, TX. The author also acknowledges Suzan Alharb.

Poster Presentation by Alison Drummond

Cell Constructs I, LLC

Innovative Antimicrobial, Regenerative Blast-Injury Therapy

Alison Drummond, Cell Constructs I, LLC
Alexander MacDougall, M.S., Cell Constructs I, LLC
Thomas Barrows, Ph.D., Cell Constructs I, LLC

Effective infection prevention combined with regenerative therapies are difficult to achieve in settings where access to medical care is delayed. There remains an unmet need to provide an integrated therapy for blast burn injuries that simultaneously delivers nonantibiotic and noncytotoxic infection prevention and healing properties. We propose an easily deployable, inexpensive solution combining the slow release of an antimicrobial compound through a permeable burn-contacting biomaterial. The burn-contacting surface is a highly biocompatible layer of human keratin protein previously shown to modulate inflammation and accelerate healing. The antimicrobial compound, N-acetyl-L-cysteine (NAC), is a noncytotoxic antioxidant which is safe, effective, and soluble in burn exudate. Our technology utilizes even minimal exudate from the burn to trigger the controlled release of NAC into the wound bed at a sustained effective dose. In acknowledgement of the austere realities of conflict zones where access to medical care can be delayed for several days, our device will have the capacity to deliver a continual effective amount for 7+ days.

The proposed solution combines (a) a nonadherent wound contacting layer composed of a proprietary subset of human keratin proteins proven to accelerate healing through several mechanisms: accelerated regranulation and reepithelialization, keratinocyte proliferation and migration, modulation of inflammation, and maintenance of a moist wound healing environment which may reduce pain; and (b) a proprietary blended layer composed of a hydrophobic, medical grade elastomer, a sparingly water-soluble, pharmaceutically acceptable plasticizer and the hydrophilic infection control agent NAC, covered with (c) a thin occlusive layer of hydrophobic elastomer. The blended layer control releases the antimicrobial agent NAC through the permeable keratin layer at a controlled rate for 7+ days upon exposure to burn exudate.

Substantial scientific evidence suggests that NAC is an ideal compound to prevent infection. In addition to being antimicrobial, NAC eliminates and prevents bacterial biofilm, a factor contributing to infection severity. In vitro testing and literature confirm effectiveness against common burn bacteria, fungi and yeast. It is an antioxidant and has its own therapeutic attributes, including an anti-inflammatory effect. Challenges of NAC include its high water solubility and resulting high concentration needed for efficacy. These challenges are resolved through the proprietary blended NAC-releasing layer of the proposed device, which provides infection protection for 7+ days. Our hypothesis is that such composition, bonded to a permeable human keratin protein burn contact layer, will prevent infection and promote healing for 7+ days.

The innovation resides within our proprietary discovery of a plasticized elastomer enabling controlled release of the nonantibiotic, hydrophilic antimicrobial NAC in a regenerative dressing format, and which does not promote drug resistant bacteria. The design focuses on simple prolonged field care, rapid application, and long term storage at ambient conditions. We hypothesize that additional hydrophilic substances, including pain relievers and hemostatic agents, will be deliverable through the same mechanism. This technology will bring a life-saving field treatment modality to the point of injury by managing infection risk and promoting healing for 7+ days before acute medical care becomes accessible.

Poster Presentation by Giorgio Giatsidis

Wound Healing Research Unit, Division of Dermatology, School of Medicine, University of Pisa

Treating Blast-Related Burns with Fluorescent Light Energy

Giorgio Giatsidis, M.D., Ph.D., Department of Surgery, Brigham and Women's Hospital
Marco Romanelli, M.D., Wound Healing Research Unit, Division of Dermatology, University of Pisa
Luc Teot, M.D., Department of Plastic and Reconstructive Surgery and Wound Healing, Lapeyronie University Hospital
Elia Ricci, M.D., Difficult Wound Healing Center, St. Luca's Clinic
Daniele Bollero, M.D., Chirurgia Plastica Piemonte
Lise Hebert, Ph.D., Klox Technologies, Inc.

Blast-related burns are among the most common injuries suffered on the battlefield. Yet, their clinical management, both acutely during evacuation and sub-acutely once wounded warriors arrive in the homeland, is still challenging and only partially effective. These complex wounds present a multifactorial disruption of several key biological processes, causing wound progression (conversion) rather than healing. Current therapeutic approaches are often able to address and correct only one or at most a limited few of these processes: as a consequence, either several pivotal biological processes are not targeted, or multiple therapies need to be combined in an empirical manner—if possible.

Fluorescent Light Energy (FLE) therapy has been shown to non-invasively and effectively modulate all the biological processes involved in wound/burn healing in an integrated manner. These include inflammation, angiogenesis, oxidative stress, bacterial growth/infection, and cell proliferation among others. The FLE System consists of a blue light-emitting diode (LED) lamp and a chromophore-containing gel. Upon illumination, the gel generates FLE that stimulates biological cascades associated with improved healing. This system allows for rapid, easy to implement, advanced care both during patient evacuation and then during sub-acute patient care.

In our preliminary experience using FLE on acute and chronic wounds, application of the gel with illumination for 5 minutes twice weekly, resulted in reduced inflammation, faster re-epithelization and wound closure, better organized collagen deposition and remodeling with improved scarring, a low rate of infections and wound breakdown, and a significant improvement in quality of life (including pain). In addition, a pilot study investigating the safety and effects of FLE in 10 patients with 2° burn injuries, showed a 100% healing rate without the need of additional skin grafting. No infection occurred during treatment.

These results suggest FLE could be a novel, simple, and safe alternative and non-invasive adjunct therapeutic solution to the standard of care for blast-related burn injuries. FLE may significantly reduce healing-time, risk of infections and complications, and pathological scarring, allowing a quicker return to pre-injury level of health and activity.

Poster Presentation by Jennifer Neff

Allvivo Vascular

Antimicrobial Peptide Formulations for Burn Wound Protection

Jennifer Neff, Ph.D., Allvivo Vascular
Danir Bayramov, Ph.D., Allvivo Vascular
Esha Patel, M.S., Allvivo Vascular
Jing Miao, M.S., Allvivo Vascular

Background: Burn wounds are a frequent component of blast injury and are prone to bacterial colonization with increased potential for invasive infection due to immune dysfunction. In prolonged evacuation scenarios, there is a need for topical antimicrobial therapies to protect burn wounds from further contamination and to control bacteria proliferation and biofilm formation. The goal of this work was to develop chitosan based formulations of an engineered antimicrobial peptide, ASP-2, and assess their capacity to eradicate biofilm associated bacteria using in vitro and ex vivo porcine skin models. The impact of replacing the levorotatory (L) form amino acids in ASP-2 with the more protease resistant dextrorotatory (D) form amino acids on peptide activity was also evaluated.

Materials and Methods: Chitosan formulations loaded with 1% ASP-2 in either D or L form were prepared in both gel and lyophilized sponge form. Peptide release from formulations was measured by reversed-phase high-performance liquid chromatography (RP-HPLC) over 7 days. Using in vitro and ex vivo porcine skin biofilm models, the efficacy of each formulation was tested against established biofilms of *Staphylococcus aureus*, *Pseudomonas aeruginosa*, and *Acinetobacter baumannii*. The activities of D and L form peptides alone were also compared using a standard minimum biocidal concentration assay.

Results: Using the chitosan formulation, 70–80% of the peptide load was released over 7 days. Chitosan formulations resulted in 3–8 log reductions in both gram positive and gram negative, drug resistant biofilm bacteria in both the in vitro and ex vivo models. Similar activities were observed between the gel and sponge formulations with improved handling observed for the sponge. Under the conditions tested, no meaningful differences in peptide activity between the L and D forms of ASP-2 were detected.

Conclusions: Chitosan based formulations provide an effective delivery platform for the engineered cationic antimicrobial peptide, ASP-2. Peptide loaded formulations are highly active against biofilms formed by both gram positive and gram negative, drug resistant bacteria relevant to burns and merit further study as a potential treatment to protect burn and other blast related wounds during prolonged evacuation.

Disclaimer: This work is supported in part by NIH NIAID Grant 1R43AI136195-01A1.

Poster Presentation by Lt Col Steven Jeffery

Royal Centre for Defence Medicine, Birmingham, United Kingdom

Kerecis (Fish Skin) for the Temporary Treatment of Burns
Lt Col Steven Jeffery, M.D., Royal Centre for Defence Medicine, Birmingham, United Kingdom

Burn excision is the gold standard treatment for full thickness and some deep partial thickness burns.

The shift towards early burn excision occurred in the 1970s, when it was shown that early burn excision improved patient outcomes. A long list of benefits have been subsequently demonstrated, including reduction in pain/length of stay/number of procedures required, quicker healing, decreased incidence of hypertrophic scarring/wound sepsis, reduced need for antibiotics, and a 3-fold decrease in mortality rate. Inflammatory mediators produced from the burn eschar can cause a systemic inflammatory response. Early burn excision in mice has shown to improve the immune system by restoring cytotoxic lymphocyte function. Overall, early burn excision maintains the immune system to fight infection and suppresses pro-inflammatory cytokine production. Early excision reduces common complications like sepsis, multi-organ failure and acute kidney injury.

"Early" has been defined as 24–96 hours after burn injury. Most surgeons perform excision on days one or two post burn injury. Excisions within 72 hours of injury using autograft have been deemed effective at treating burn injury. Therefore, excision within 72 hours should be the goal when treating full thickness burns, even in a mass casualty scenario.

When treating large burns, autologous skin availability becomes a problem and burn surgeons often rely heavily on allogenic and xenogeneic skin for temporary coverage after excision. Human cadaver and pig skin are major sources of this temporary coverage. Cadaveric skin is in limited supply and requires a logistic chain unsuited to use in the field. Pig skin is required to be stored frozen, and the supply is also limited.

There has recently become available an alternative resource of xenograft using acellular fish skin (KerecisTM Omega3 Burn). This has been described as providing an effective, safe, efficient skin substitute, free of the risk of transmission of viral disease and auto-immune reaction risk.

The fish skin is stored at room temperature, has a shelf life of three years and is marketed as an off-the-shelf product. Due to these properties, fish skin is an ideal choice for the treatment of combat casualties at the Field Hospital level, where cadaver skin or pig skin are not practical to use due to their short shelf life and cold chain issues. As a byproduct of the fishing industry, the amount of fish skin that could be produced and stored is potentially extremely large. Large amounts of the product could rapidly be transported to the area of need, thereby allowing for the correct management of burn injury despite having a large number of casualties.

Kerecis has already been extensively tested on pigs and has also been used in humans for both partial thickness and full thickness burns. An randomized controlled trial (RCT) is currently ongoing comparing Kerecis with cadaveric allograft in treatment for full thickness burns at MedStar Health Research Institute, Washington, D.C. The results of preclinical studies have demonstrated that the fish skin is as good as cadaver skin for temporary coverage and furthermore, that by using it with highly meshed split-thickness skin graft (STSG) leads to significant reduction in STSG requirements.

Poster Presentation by Aprile L. Pilon

APCBio Innovations, Inc.

Comparative CC10 Effects in Inhalation +/– Burn Injuries

Aprile L. Pilon, Ph.D., APCBio Innovations, Inc.
Richard S. Clayton, M.S., APCBio Innovations, Inc.
Melissa E. Winn, B.S., APCBio Innovations, Inc.
Ernesto Lopez, M.D., Ph.D., University of Texas Medical Branch
Pereniel Enkhbaatar, M.D., Ph.D., University of Texas Medical Branch

Blast-induced injuries often include a combination of burn and inhalation injuries. Recombinant human club cell 10 kDa protein (rhCC10) has previously been shown to decrease airway inflammation in several animal models of acute lung injury and in human neonates with respiratory distress of prematurity. We evaluated the effects of rhCC10 in an ovine model of traumatic smoke inhalation with and without dermal burn. Smoke inhalation injury was induced in adult female ewes by cotton smoke insufflation with or without third degree burns to 40% total body surface area. After injury, sheep were placed on mechanical ventilation with analgesia. Treatment with intravenous rhCC10 (1, 3, or 10 mg/kg/day) or vehicle was initiated one hour after injury with repeat doses every 12 hours. A total of 30 animals were evaluated for smoke inhalation only (SO), 22 for smoke plus burn (B+S), and 3 for burn only (BO). An additional 6 sham animals were instrumented but not injured. Animals were euthanized 48 hours after injury. Overall, rhCC10 had similar effects on several physiologic measures in SO and B+S at 48, but there were differences, including the severity of pulmonary inflammation and pharmacokinetics. Lung tissue myeloperoxidase (MPO) activity was significantly elevated in SO compared to sham but was not elevated in B+S. RhCC10 treatment reduced MPO activity in lung tissue close to baseline/sham levels ($p = 0.05$) in SO. However, since lung MPO activity was not different than sham in the B+S injury, rhCC10 did not reduce MPO in B+S injury. The bioavailability of rhCC10 was also altered in the B+S compared to SO. The mean maximum value and range for plasma CC10 was reduced ~1.5X in B+S compared to smoke only, despite that there was no difference in the circulating half-life. Most importantly, treatment with IV 10 mg/kg/day rhCC10 improved survival in SO and B+S injuries and we have recently identified a novel pathway through which rhCC10 may mediate its effects in SO and B+S injuries. Thus, rhCC10 is a promising therapeutic for treatment of smoke inhalation injury with and without dermal burns.

Disclaimer: Research funded in part by DoD grant W81XWH-12-1-0514 to ALP at Therabron Therapeutics, a predecessor of APCBio Innovations, Inc.

Poster Presentation by David Peralta

BlueWillow Biologics

Topical Nanoemulsion Therapy for Burn Wound Progression
David Peralta, B.B.A., BlueWillow Biologics
Mark Hemmila, M.D., University of Michigan Trauma Burn Center
Susan Ciotti, Ph.D., BlueWillow Biologics
David Muth, BlueWillow Biologics

Burn injury is one of the most common and devastating forms of trauma. 100,000 patients suffer moderate to severe burn injuries requiring hospitalization each year, of these cases about 5,000 patients die from burn-related complications. Burn wound progression is a process by which an initial partial-thickness burn injury can advance to a deep partial-thickness or full-thickness burn wound. The cause of burn wound progression is multifactorial but depends on a component of the host response and inflammation. Progression of the initial burn injury towards increased tissue damage is an important phenomenon due to the fact that burn wound depth is the principal determinant of morbidity and the need for surgical treatment. A partial-thickness burn wound which does not progress to full-thickness is capable of self-healing. The skin regenerates from the undamaged epithelial cells that line the shaft of each hair follicle. However, progression to deep partial-thickness or a full-thickness burn wound requires intensive surgical treatment such as operative excision of the dead tissue and skin grafting to restore the patient's skin integrity. This is a painful, labor intensive process that can require many weeks or months of costly hospitalization. In addition, the patient is permanently disfigured and may have long term problems with the reconstructed skin as it is never the same as the original. Development of a topical therapy that halts burn wound progression while acting as a topical antimicrobial would be a significant breakthrough in the treatment of thermal burn injury. It would lessen the need for skin grafting, speed recovery, result in fewer infectious complications, and improve the outcomes for many burn patients. In a rodent model, we have used a novel antimicrobial nanoemulsion to treat burn injured skin. The nanoemulsion reduces bacterial growth in the burn wound to minimal levels, significantly reduces excess inflammation and reduces pain scores. By reducing excess influx of neutrophils into the burn wound and modulating the pro-inflammatory response the nanoemulsion compound appears to diminish burn wound progression in the early post-injury phase. We have conducted additional studies in a Porcine (pig) wound model which again shows the effectiveness of topically applied anti-microbial nanoemulsion on abating burn wound progression, promoting wound healing, acting as an effective anti-microbial, and assessing for acute toxicity. The porcine (pig) burn wound model, is an optimal in-vivo vehicle for assessing burn wound progression as it mimics human skin more closely than the rodent model we have utilized in our prior investigative work. The development of a novel antimicrobial and inflammatory modulating topical therapy for early burn wound treatment to thwart conversion of partial-thickness burns to full-thickness injury due to progression of the thermal injury would revolutionize treatment for soldiers who experience burn injuries in the field.

Poster Presentation by Kenneth A. Gruber

Tensive Controls

Symptoms of Burn Injury vs. Cachexia: Two Terms-One Syndrome
Kenneth A. Gruber, Ph.D., Tensive Controls
Michael F. Callahan, Ph.D., Tensive Controls
Jessica Newton Northup, M.S., Tensive Controls

Burn trauma presents unique treatment problems when it occurs in small combat units in austere environments, especially when there is delayed evacuation to a higher medical care echelon. Systemic symptoms include hypermetabolism and a catabolic physiological state; which produces protein/caloric malnutrition, immune suppression and infection. These symptoms contribute to sepsis, and delayed wound healing and recovery. Tensive Controls (TCI) has a drug candidate that potentially addresses many of these symptoms.

There are many similarities between burns and disease-induced cachexia; e.g. loss of body weight (BW), multiorgan failure, and breakdown of the intestinal barrier. These effects appear to be proinflammatory cytokine-dependent. Reports of burn injuries often note BW loss as a cachexia symptom. However, a link between the systemic effects of cachexia and burns (e.g., multiorgan failure) was not appreciated.

Over the past 15 years, the discovery that the melanocortin (MC) system regulates metabolism led to the successful use of CNS administered MC-4 receptor (MC4R) antagonists in the alleviation of experimental disease-induced cachexia, as well as acute radiation syndrome.

MC4R antagonists must cross the blood brain barrier (BBB) to reach the metabolism controlling MC4Rs. In order to overcome this "access" problem, TCI developed a platform technology to produce actively transported drug-like peptides. This eventually resulted in TCMCB07, a MC4R antagonist with BBB transport properties.

TCMCB07 increased BW in rat cachexia due to cancer, bacterial toxins, or uremia. However, in drug development, the translational efficiency of rodent to human is 90%; i.e., the dog is a superior model for developing drugs. To take advantage of this relationship, TCI developed a canine cachexia veterinary hospitals' trials network to test TCMCB07.

TCMCB07 reversed life-threatening cachexia in an "all comers" trial in dogs. Currently 12 dogs have completed the 4-week trial, including 4 on expanded access. Prior to trial, cachectic dogs had lost an average of 5–10% BW. This reversed to a 6% BW gain on the drug. Of these dogs, 4 were minimal responders, BWs merely stabilized; a 75% response rate. In the 12 dogs, there were no reports of significant side effects, even in those on the drug for hundreds of days.

TCMCB07 is a potential therapeutic/prophylactic for cachexia-like burn symptoms, easily administered in a field situation, and potentially incorporated into a military medic kit or a soldier's individual first aid kit. TCMCB07 is entering the safety-toxicology tests required for FDA Investigational New Drug (IND) approval.

Poster Presentation by Augustine Chuang

Eisenhower Army Medical Center

Effective Treatment on In Vitro Blast-Burn Models

Augustine Chuang, Ph.D., Eisenhower Army Medical Center
Jeremy L. Goodin, Ph.D., Eisenhower Army Medical Center
James C. McPherson III, Ph.D., Eisenhower Army Medical Center

We developed an in vitro Wound Healing Model to evaluate blast injury response and wound repopulation (healing) over time in hard/soft tissues. The data yielded a damaged tissue dose response curve to blast pressure and a significant difference in wound healing over time. An increased blast pressure at the tissue culture face (30.0 psi) yielded significant increases in cell repopulation of the wound over time (from 8% at day two to 88% at day eight), but significantly lower than non-blast controls (13% to 96% wound repopulation). As expected, a lower blast pressure (19.47 psi) yielded wound repopulation rates from 6% on day two to 95% on day eight with non-blast controls yielding 14% to 98%, and not significantly different by day two. In in vivo rat third degree burn studies, we administered IV Pluronic F-127 30 min post-burn, yielding a significant reduction in wound contraction and histologically less microscopic damage associated with full thickness burns at 48 hrs. There was a significant improvement in closure rates of treated rats at 30 days. In rat thermal paw edema studies, Pluronic F-68 significantly prevented or blunted the edema response to thermal injury when given before or 30 min after injury, respectively. We propose the use of our wound healing model on hard/soft tissue cultures subjected to a blast injury and followed immediately by the addition of media and incubation at elevated temperatures to evaluate treatment modalities yielding significant improvement in wound repopulation and repair. We currently assess this evaluation by following Live/Dead Cell Assay results, % wound repopulation, and the measures of cytokines and cell markers in culture media and cell lysate over time, resulting in positive therapeutic treatments.

Poster Presentation by Nicusor Iftimia

Physical Sciences Inc.

Hand-Held Probe for Noninvasive Assessment of Burn Injuries

Nicusor Iftimia, Ph.D., Physical Sciences Inc.
Jesung Park, Ph.D., Physical Sciences Inc.
Robert Sheridan, Ph.D., Shriners Hospital

Skin injuries, particularly skin burns, are an omnipresent threat in the military environment. With the ever-increasing destructive power and efficiency of modern weapons, casualties—both fatal and non-fatal—are reaching new highs, among both civilians and military personnel. Most injuries heal on their own, but complex wounds warrant a specialist and skilled multidisciplinary approach for a successful clinical outcome. Among skin injuries, burns are the most difficult to treat. Burn wounds are dynamic and need reassessment in the first 24–72 hours because depth can increase as a result of inadequate treatment or superadded infection. A critical part of burn management is assessing the depth and the extent of the injury. Usually, the assessment is done visually, and can be very subjective, depending on clinician's training and years of experience. Clinical examination alone is not always sufficient to determine which burn wounds will heal spontaneously and which will require surgical intervention for optimal outcome, and even more importantly, why a wound that was initially assessed as properly healing fails to heal. Therefore, it is critical for a burn specialist to have the adequate tools for objective assessment of the wound healing status.

To address this issue, Physical Sciences Inc., in collaboration with Shriners Hospital developed an optical imaging tool for more objective diagnosing of skin wounds and for evaluating healing prospects after injury. Our approach is to investigate the simultaneous use of two high-resolution imaging technologies, reflectance confocal microscopy (RCM) and optical coherence tomography (OCT), for assessing skin injury gravity and determine the right therapy regimen to prevent severe inflammation following injury and thus to prevent subsequent injury progression. These two optical technologies have complementary capabilities that can offer the clinician a set of clinically comprehensive parameters: OCT helps to visualize morphological and functional changes on both layers of the skin and thus examine important imaging biomarkers such as inflammation, scarring, vascular extravasation, wound depth, and collagen integrity, while RCM provides submicron details (sub-cellular resolution) of the epidermal layer and upper dermis, and thus helps to visualize subcellular biomarkers such as cell inflammation or damage, as well as blood flow in the upper dermis. Preliminary evaluation of this technology on over 20 skin burn patients has demonstrated its capability to objectively assess injury status and monitor therapy progress. Therefore, we strongly believe that this technology could help clinicians in the future to more reliably diagnose burn lesions and objectively assess healing prospects.

Poster Presentation by Elaine Christine MacAslan

Cornerstone Research Group, Inc.

Magnetic Analgesia Cuff
Elaine Christine MacAslan, Cornerstone Research Group, Inc.

Burns add significant complexity to medical care and decrease the overall likelihood of survival of a multitrauma injury such as a blast injury. Pain management in the burn patient is a severe challenge and inappropriate analgesic treatment is a continuing, common issue. The primary means of treating pain in burn patients is drug administration. However, decreased blood flow during the initial inflammatory response and later capillary leakage result in altered pharmacokinetics. Furthermore, delay is an inherent disadvantage of pharmacological pain management, complicating dressing changes, patient movement, and other critical aspects of care. Inadequate pain control results in suffering, diminished trust in the medical team, and potentially the development of chronic pain and posttraumatic stress disorder.

The perception of pain relies on nociceptive fibers conducting action potentials (APs) from the injury to the brain. Lidocaine (for example) can be used intravenously to manage neuropathic pain. By binding to ion channels, it inhibits the movement of sodium ions into nerve cells and blocks axons from conducting APs. Blocking these APs results in analgesia.

Cornerstone Research Group, Inc. (CRG) is developing the Quick Magnetic Analgesia Cuff (QMAC), an externally wearable, non-invasive, battery-operated device capable of providing analgesia equivalent to pharmacological peripheral ring nerve blocks by manipulating axonal activity with magnetic fields. CRG's device will also block APs, but it will use a magnetic field instead of molecular binding to do so. Magnetic fields induce electric currents in conductive materials, such as neuronal axons. These induced currents may depolarize or hyperpolarize the axonal membrane, blocking the conduction of APs. Blocking these APs results in analgesia distal to the block. By generating a magnetic field suitable for depolarizing or hyperpolarizing nociceptive fibers, the QMAC would provide analgesia. CRG is currently in the early stages of the project and designing the magnetic coils to apply the electric field of interest.

This approach enables on-demand analgesia, facilitating pain management and medical care. It also minimizes challenges associated with drugs, such as diversion, overdose, allergic reactions, paresthesia, and risk of addiction. In particular, the QMAC is suitable for prolonged field care in that it is simple to use and requires no available pharmacological agents or sterile injection supplies.

Disclaimer: This work is funded by the Defense Health Agency (DHA).

Poster Presentation by Lt Col Steven Jeffery

Royal Centre for Defence Medicine, Birmingham, United Kingdom

Sprayable Topical Anaesthetics for Burn-Related Injury

Lt Col Steven Jeffery, M.D., Royal Centre for Defence Medicine, Birmingham, United Kingdom

Blast-related burn injuries are typically a combination of superficial 'flash' burns where skin has been directly exposed to a very high temperature for a very short period of time, together with deeper burns where clothing has caught fire causing full thickness burns to the underlying skin.

Superficial burns are very painful, as the nerve endings are not only intact but directly exposed to the air. This pain is usually treated with opioid analgesia, via intravenous injection of morphine, or by the use of an oral transmucosal fentanyl citrate (OTFC) lozenge, which is issued to deployed military personnel. Side effects of opioids include respiratory depression (which may lead to an increased reliance on airway support), and constriction of the pupils, resulting in visual impairment and interfering with the diagnosis of a concomitant head injury, as well as interfering with the ability to continue fighting. The storage and issuing of opioids to the public are also problematic because of the potential for mis-use.

In the veterinary market a product called Tri-Solfen® (Animal Ethics Pty Ltd Melbourne Australia) has been available to veterinarians in the Southern Hemisphere for many years which provides topical multi-modal anaesthesia for animals with painful wounds (including superficial and full thickness burns). This product contains a mixture of short acting (lidocaine) and long acting (bupivacaine) local anaesthetics together with adrenaline (to reduce bleeding) and cetrimide (a proven antiseptic agent). This product is designed to 'spray and stay' i.e. stick to the wound surface once sprayed on, providing a barrier over the exposed nerve endings and prolonged contact with the local anaesthetics. Only a little product is therefore required to give instant and long-lasting pain relief.

Work is ongoing to bring this concept of sprayable topical anaesthetics combined with two other components for wounds to the human market. Currently first-in-man trials are underway in the UK ensuring that the safety and levels of efficacy of the product meet the appropriate regulatory requirements.

If early trials are successful, it is envisaged that the availability of this product could allow for safe, fast acting and long-lasting pain relief in large numbers of casualties with blast-related burn injury, and/or have an opiate-sparing action. Deployed military personnel could be issued with a small ruggedized canister containing the solution instead of/as well as the OTFC.

Other potential benefits from the early application of the antiseptic agent, are also being studied. We aim to describe progress with our research strategy and look for partners to help bring this potentially innovative and effective product to market for human use, in blast-injury casualty settings.

Poster Presentation by Jeffrey Colombe

MITRE Corporation

MHS Blast Injury Prevention Standard for Dermal Burns and the Science of Burn Injury Risk to the Dermis from Explosive Blasts and Secondary Conflagrations

Jeffrey Colombe, Ph.D., MITRE Corporation
Brian Colder, Ph.D., MITRE Corporation
Jennifer Lombardo, B.S., MITRE Corporation
Rachel Spencer, RN, MHSA, MITRE Corporation
Lisa Lalis, B.S., MITRE Corporation

The MHS Blast Injury Prevention Standards Recommendation (BIPSR) Process was established to identify and meticulously evaluate the details of existing blast injury prevention standards to determine suitability for use by the DoD in health hazard assessments to design safe weapon systems, crew survivability assessments to build survivable combat vehicles, and the design and testing of protective systems. It evaluates the suitability of existing candidate standards to meet DoD Stakeholder requirements. Following the steps of the BIPSR Process, the Dermal Burns Blast Injury Type was initiated with survey of the current state of science on burn injury risk to the dermis from explosive blasts and secondary conflagrations, including a literature survey and interview with subject matter experts, undertaken to identify candidate injury risk criteria for potential recommendation as MHS Blast Injury Prevention Standards.

These early activities of the BIPSR Process revealed military and civilian standards for burn injury prevention already in use, although none identified so far specify blast hazards. Most burn injury prevention standards reviewed are intended to experimentally measure the reduction in heat transfer from thermally protective garments in highly controlled laboratory environments. Protocols for test and evaluation of such garments are based on comparisons between heat sensor readings on 'naked' manikins versus those wearing protective garments, resulting in an estimate of the relative reduction in heat transfer to skin provided by garments.

The estimation of injury risk to tissue involves a modeling and simulation approach for assessing injury based on a given temporal pattern of heat transfer to skin. Such methods use an experimentally derived theoretical model of tissue injury as a function of heat transfer. The approach is based on the Arrhenius equation, which is ordinarily used to calculate activation energy of chemical reactions. In the case of dermal burns, the chemical reactions remain unspecified, but correspond phenomenologically to denaturation of proteins and rupture of cell membranes, among other potential tissue changes (Despa et al., 2005). Burn prediction uses a time integral of instantaneous tissue damage as a function of temperature above 44 degrees Celsius (111 degrees Fahrenheit; Moritz and Henriques, 1947), increasing logarithmically with temperature, fit to data from human and porcine experimental tests. The dominant instantiation of the approach is the BURNSIM model (Knox, 1979; Knox, Bonetti, and Perry, 1993) and refinements of this model, which simulate heat transfer through the spatial extent of skin using finite difference voxels in a lattice. Heat flows from its source through tissue over time using a Fourier heat conduction calculation, and burns are predicted when the local damage integral crosses an experimentally determined threshold. Recent work has extended these threshold-based injury prediction models to more general statistical injury risk curves that indicate the sample population likelihood of burns of varying severity based on temporally integrated instantaneous tissue damage (Iyoho, Ng, and Chan, 2017).

Once the current landscape is well understood, next steps in the BIPSR Process include engagement with DoD Stakeholders to understand how they would use an MHS Dermal Burns Blast Injury Prevention Standard.

Disclaimer: The opinions and assertions contained herein are the private views of the author and are not to be construed as official or reflecting the views of the Department of the Army or the Department of Defense. This technical data deliverable was developed using contract funds under Basic Contract No. W56KGU-18-C-0010. Approved for Public Release, Distribution Unlimited. 19-3476 © The MITRE Corporation

Previous State-of-the-Science Meetings

1. International State-of-the-Science Meeting on Non-Impact, Blast-Induced Mild Traumatic Brain Injury, May 12–14, 2009, in Herndon, Va.
https://blastinjuryresearch.amedd.army.mil/assets/docs/sos/meeting_proceedings/2009_SoS_Meeting_Proceedings.pdf

2. International State-of-the-Science Meeting on Blast Injury Dosimetry, June 8–10, 2010, in Chantilly, Va.
https://blastinjuryresearch.amedd.army.mil/assets/docs/sos/meeting_proceedings/2010_SoS_Meeting_Proceedings.pdf

3. International State-of-the-Science Meeting on Blast-Induced Tinnitus, November 15–17, 2011, in Chantilly, Va.
https://blastinjuryresearch.amedd.army.mil/assets/docs/sos/meeting_proceedings/2011_SoS_Meeting_Proceedings.pdf

4. International State-of-the-Science Meeting on the Biomedical Basis for Mild Traumatic Brain Injury Environmental Sensor Threshold Values, November 4–6, 2014, in McLean, Va.
https://blastinjuryresearch.amedd.army.mil/assets/docs/sos/meeting_proceedings/2014_SoS_Meeting_Proceedings.pdf

5. International State-of-the-Science Meeting: Does Repeated Blast-Related Trauma Contribute to the Development of Chronic Traumatic Encephalopathy? November 3–5, 2015, in McLean, Va.
https://blastinjuryresearch.amedd.army.mil/assets/docs/sos/meeting_proceedings/2015_SoS_Meeting_Proceedings.pdf

6. International State-of-the-Science Meeting on Minimizing the Impact of Wound Infections Following Blast-Related Injuries, November 29–December 1, 2016, in Arlington, Va.
https://blastinjuryresearch.amedd.army.mil/assets/docs/sos/meeting_proceedings/2016_SoS_Meeting_Proceedings.pdf

7. International State-of-the-Science Meeting on the Neurological Effects of Repeated Exposure to Military Occupational Blast: Implications for Prevention and Health, March 12–15, 2018, in Arlington, Va.
https://www.rand.org/pubs/conf_proceedings/CF380z1.html

8. International State-of-the-Science Meeting on Limb Salvage and Recovery After Blast-Related Injury, March 5–8, 2020, in Arlington, Va.
https://www.rand.org/pubs/conf_proceedings/CF420.html

Agenda of the Ninth State-of-the-Science Meeting

Day 1: Tuesday, March 3, 2020

Time	Schedule	Presenter
7:30	Registration Opens	
8:00	*Welcome from the Acting Director, Department of Defense Blast Injury Research Coordinating Office*	Dr. Raj Gupta
8:10	*Welcome from the Acting Principal Assistant for Research and Technology, U.S. Army Medical Research and Development Command*	Dr. Mark Dertzbaugh
8:25	*Brief Meeting Overview*	Dr. Charles C. Engel
8:35	*Keynote Address: Military Burn Care: Tales from the Leading Edge of Innovation*	COL Kevin K. Chung, M.D, U.S. Army
9:05	*Invited Presentations, Session One*	Expert panelist, Dr. Matthias Donelan
9:05	Blast-Related Burns: A Modern History	Dr. Leopoldo C. Cancio
9:25	Overview of DoD Burn Research	Dr. Kai Leung
9:45	Military Health System Burn Injury Prevention Standard: Example of Dermal Burn Science	Dr. Jeffrey Colombe
10:05	*Q&A Panel*	*(Cancio, Leung, Colombe)*
10:20	*AM BREAK*	
10:40	*Invited Presentations, Session Two*	Expert panelist, Dr. Narayan Iyer
10:40	Civilian Burn Mass Casualty Events and Preparedness Research	Dr. Colleen Ryan
11:00	Prehospital Burn Care: Prolonged Field Care	COL Jeremy Pamplin, M.D., U.S. Army
11:20	Acute Assessment and Management of Burn Injury	Dr. Eileen Bulger
11:40	Impact of Acute Care on Long Term Outcomes	Dr. Nicole S. Gibran
12:00	*Q&A Panel*	*(Ryan, Pamplin, Bulger, Gibran)*
12:15	*LUNCH AND POSTER SETUP*	
1:30	*Invited Presentations, Session Three*	Expert panelist, Dr. Nicole S. Gibran
1:30	Surgical Advances: Reconstruction and Restoration	Dr. Rodney Chan
1:50	Psychosocial Aspects of Resilience and Functioning	Dr. Amanda Reichard
2:10	RAND Literature Review Summary	Dr. Tepring Piquado
2:30	*Q&A Panel*	*(Chan, Reichard, Piquado)*
2:45	*PM BREAK*	
3:00	*Scientific Presentations, Session One: Populations and Planning*	Expert panelist, Dr. Leopoldo C. Cancio
3:00	Burn Injuries in U.S. Service Members: 2001–2018	Katheryne Perez
3:15	U.S. Army Burn Center Registry and Burn Injury Model System	Dr. Radha K. Holavanahalli
3:30	TBI, Burns and Blast: Is PTSD All About the Blast?	Dr. Mary Jo Pugh
3:45	National Trauma Research Action Plan: A Burn Research Agenda	Dr. Nicole S. Gibran
4:00	*Q&A Panel*	*(Perez, Holavanahalli, Pugh, Gibran)*

Time	Schedule	Presenter
4:15	*Closing Remarks*	Dr. Raj Gupta Dr. Charles C. Engel
4:30	*Adjourn*	

Day 2: Wednesday, March 4, 2020

Time	Schedule	Presenter
7:00	Registration Opens	
8:00	*Welcome*	Dr. Raj Gupta
8:10	*Scientific Presentations Two: Injury Assessment and Technology*	Expert panelist, Dr. Amanda Reichard
8:10	A Warrior Avatar for Model Based Blast and Burn Injury	Dr. H. T. Garimella
8:25	In Vivo Terahertz Spectral Imaging for Burn Depth Diagnosis	Dr. M. Hassan Arbab
8:40	Creating an Automated, Enhanced Lund Browder Diagram to Calculate TBSA	Gregory T. Rule
8:55	Blood mRNA Integrity Is a Marker of Radiation Exposure	Dr. Lauren Moffatt
9:10	*Speaker Q&As*	*(Garimella, Arbab, Rule, Moffatt)*
9:25	*AM BREAK*	
9:40	*Scientific Presentations Three: Intervention Research*	Expert panelist, Dr. William Scott Dewey
9:40	Burn Resuscitation: Can We Be Better?	Dr. Jeanne Lee
9:55	Nanofiber Dressings for Infection Prevention and Pain Relief	Dr. Jessica Amber Jennings
10:10	*Speaker Q&As*	*(Lee, Jennings)*
10:55	*Work Group Roles and Responsibilities*	*Emily Hoch*
11:15	*LUNCH AND POSTERS*	
12:30	Break out to work groups*	Expert panelists
4:00	*Adjourn directly from work groups*	

*Breaks are determined within each work group.

Day 3: Thursday, March 5, 2020

Time	Schedule	Presenter
7:00	Registration	
8:00	Reconvene in work groups*	
10:00	*Work Group Reports*	Dr. Charles C. Engel, moderator
10:00	Work Group A: Dr. Leopoldo C. Cancio** Room 4206	
10:15	Work Group B: Dr. Nicole S. Gibran** Room 4204	
10:30	Work Group C: Dr. Narayan Iyer** Room 4306	
10:45	Work Group D: Dr. Matthias Donelan** Room 4200	
11:00	Work Group E: Dr. William Scott Dewey** Room 4232	
11:15	Work Group F: Dr. Amanda Reichard** Room 4128	
11:30	*Speaker Q&As*	
12:00	*Closing Remarks and Adjourn*	Dr. Raj Gupta
12:15	*Closed Session—Expert Panel*	*(Cancio, Dewey, Donelan, Gibran, Iyer, Reichard)*

*Breaks are determined within each work group.
**Expert panelist.

Biography of Keynote Speaker COL Kevin K. Chung

COL Kevin K. Chung is a graduate of the U.S. Military Academy at West Point and the Georgetown University School of Medicine. He is currently chair of the Department of Medicine at the Uniformed Services University of the Health Sciences in Bethesda, Maryland. Previously, Chung was chief of medicine at Brooke Army Medical Center in Fort Sam Houston, Texas. Prior to this, he was assigned to USAISR, where he has served in the capacity of medical director of the BICU, Task Area Manager of Clinical Trials in Burns and Trauma, and director of research for the research directorate. Chung holds academic appointments at the Uniformed Services University of the Health Sciences as a professor for both the Department of Medicine and the Department of Surgery. In 2014, he was appointed the Critical Care Consultant to the Army Surgeon General. In 2017, he was elected into the board of trustees of the ABA as the second vice president. In his career, Chung has authored 205 manuscripts in peer-reviewed journals and 18 book chapters, and he has been an invited speaker for more than 100 lectures internationally. He is also an ad hoc reviewer for ten major medical journals, including the *New England Journal of Medicine* and *Critical Care Medicine*, and is on the editorial board of *Burns*. Additionally, he is the coinventor of the Decision-Assist Method for Resuscitation, which won the Army's Greatest Invention Award. In 2013, the decision-assist algorithm was adopted into a device and approved by the FDA. Chung's research interests include combat casualty care, burns, critical care, and organ support.

Expert Panel Biographies

An expert panel of six subject-matter experts, representing policymakers, clinicians, and scientists, helped lead and focus discussions during the plenary sessions. The expert panel members also chaired working group sessions, during which participants discussed the meeting questions.

Leopoldo (Lee) C. Cancio, M.D., F.A.C.S., FCCM

Dr. Lee Cancio is the director of the U.S. Army Burn Center at USAISR in San Antonio, Texas. During his 27-year active-duty career in the U.S. Army, he deployed with the 504th Parachute Infantry Regiment of the 82nd Airborne Division to Operation Just Cause in Panama in 1989–1990 and to Operation Desert Storm in 1990–1991. While on active duty at USAISR, he served in various positions, culminating as director of the Burn Center, and established the Special Medical Augmentation Response Teams for burns. In 2003, during OIF, he deployed with U.S. Special Operations Command Central as the principal investigator in theater for the hemostatic dressing protocol. He served as the Deputy Commander for Clinical Services at the 86th Combat Support Hospital in Baghdad during OIF in 2005, and again in 2008. In 2013, he deployed with a Forward Surgical Team to Afghanistan during OEF. He retired in 2014 in the rank of colonel.

Cancio's military awards and decorations include the Legion of Merit, Bronze Star Award (one oak leaf cluster), Parachutist Badge with a combat jump star, Air Assault Badge, Expert Field Medical Badge, Combat Medical Badge, Senior Aircraft Crewman Badge, Surgeon General's "A" proficiency designator, and Order of Military Medical Merit. In 2017, he became the second civilian director and the first government civilian director of the U.S. Army Burn Center.

Cancio is a graduate of Amherst College, the Catholic University of America, and the Georgetown University School of Medicine. He completed a residency in general surgery at Brooke Army Medical Center and a fellowship in surgical critical care at the San Antonio Uniformed Services Health Education Consortium. He is board-certified in surgery and surgical critical care. Cancio's research interests include burn shock, hemorrhagic shock, acute respiratory distress syndrome, and blast injury. He established two successful research task areas within the Combat Casualty Care Research Program of the U.S. Army Medical Research and Materiel Command (Combat Critical Care Engineering and Multi-Organ Support Technology). He is the coinventor of the first commercially available decision-support system for burn-shock resuscitation, the Burn Navigator (Arcos Medical, Houston, Texas). He contributed preclinical data to the FDA approval of the ER-REBOA Catheter (Prytime Medical, Boerne, Texas). He is the author of more than 200 peer-reviewed papers, 25 chapters, and other works.

Cancio is a member of the American College of Surgeons (including the Committee on Trauma), American Association for the Surgery of Trauma, Eastern Association for the Surgery of Trauma, Shock Society, International Society for Burn Injuries, Society for Critical Care Medicine, Surgical Discovery Club, and ABA. He currently serves as the secretary of the ABA and as a member of its Verification Committee for burn centers. He is a member of the editorial boards of *Burns*, the *Journal of Burn Care & Research*, and the *American Journal of Disaster Medicine*. He is a professor of surgery (adjunct) at the University of Texas Health Science Center at San Antonio.

William Scott Dewey, PT, CHT

William Scott Dewey is a physical therapist and certified hand therapist. He has been practicing for 24 years and, for the past 16 years, has worked at the U.S. Army Burn Center in San Antonio, Texas. He currently serves as the Chief of Rehabilitation and is active in research, teaching, administration, and clinical practice. He served as the co–principal investigator of the multicenter study *A Goniometry Paradigm Shift to Measure Burn Scar Contracture in Burn Patients* (Parry and Dewey, 2019). He has also served as an investigator on multisite rehabilitation trials and a reviewer for the Congressionally Directed Medical Research Programs. He has published more than 50 articles and delivered more than 100 presentations on burn and hand rehabilitation.

Dewey holds additional certifications in advanced burn life support and degrees from the University of Texas Health Science Center and Texas A&M University.

Matthias Donelan, M.D.

Dr. Matthias Donelan is on the active medical staff in plastic surgery for Shriners Hospitals for Children in Boston, Massachusetts, and is board-certified by the American Board of Plastic Surgery. He earned an undergraduate degree in biology from Harvard College and a medical degree from the Tufts University School of Medicine. Donelan completed his residency in plastic surgery at Massachusetts General Hospital and a student fellowship in pathology at New England Medical Center in Boston.

Donelan is a widely recognized specialist in the field of burn reconstructive surgery and has developed numerous innovative techniques to enhance the care of burn patients. He has multiple publications in peer-reviewed scientific journals and has written definitive textbook chapters on burn reconstruction. Donelan has long been an advocate for scar rehabilitation through tension relief and the use of the pulsed-dye laser. He is currently investigating fractional carbon dioxide laser treatment for aesthetic and reconstructive indications in burn and trauma patients. In addition to his clinical and scientific activities, he is involved in residency training and is on the executive committee of the Harvard Combined Plastic Surgery Training Program.

Nicole S. Gibran, M.D., F.A.C.S.

Dr. Nicole S. Gibran received her bachelor's degree at Brown University and her medical degree at Boston University. After a residency in the Boston University Department of Surgery under the mentorship of Dr. Erwin Hirsch, she completed a clinical fellowship in the University of Washington Medicine Regional Burn Center with Dr. David Heimbach and Dr. Loren Engrav, followed by an NIH Trauma Research T32 fellowship. A professor in the University of Washington Medicine Department of Surgery, Gibran was the director of the University of Washington Medicine Regional Burn Center from 2002 through 2018 and the University of Washington Burn Fellowship from 2002 through 2014. In these roles, she emphasized team building and mentoring residents and junior faculty. She now serves as Associate Dean for Research and Graduate Education at the University of Washington School of Medicine.

For the past 28 years, Gibran has cared for patients with burn injuries and conducted research in the areas of burn care and response to injury. Clinically, she has been most interested in promoting optimal clinical outcomes by introducing metrics into daily practice, both in her practice and nationally. In addition to fulfilling duties in patient care and teaching, Gibran developed the University of Washington Medicine Regional Burn Center Research Laboratory with emphasis on aberrant healing processes, including hypertrophic scar formation and chronic nonhealing wounds seen with diabetes mellitus. Her research has been continually federally funded since 1997. Her basic and translational research program has encompassed responses to cutaneous injury that impact resuscitation, inflammation, wound repair, and scarring. Since 2011, Gibran has served as the program director for the Northwest Regional Burn Model System, which is funded by NIDILRR. This program has focused on improving psychological and physical quality of life for burn survivors, including identifying ways to enhance community reintegration and return to work by collecting long-term patient-reported outcomes data, disseminating information about burn injuries to individuals affected by burn injury, and promoting knowledge translation. Gibran has advocated for incorporating patient voices in burn center and national research and quality improvement programs and has encouraged the inclusion of patient-reported outcomes data in national burn registries to increase understanding of long-term patient needs. She has more than 190 publications in the areas of wound repair, responses to injury, and burn outcomes. She served on the NIH Center for Scientific Review Surgery, Anesthesiology and Trauma institutional review board (IRB) study section and was chair from 2005 to 2007.

Gibran has been a member of the ABA since 1991, serving on the Research, Program, and Ethics committees and the Committee on the Organization and Delivery of Burn Care (CODBC). While she was chair of the CODBC, her committee guided the ABA organizational policy on disaster planning for burn mass casualties. She was actively involved in establishing the Burn Fellowship guidelines. She served as ABA president from 2011 to 2012, during which she emphasized the need for the burn community to embrace outcomes measurement as part of the quest for quality and patient safety and launched the national ABA Burn Quality Improvement Program.

Currently, Gibran studies genetic and epigenetic pathophysiologic causes of fibroproliferative responses to injury. She serves on the executive committee of the National Trauma Institute and the American College of Surgeons (ACS) Committee on Trauma.

Narayan Iyer, Ph.D.

Dr. Narayan Iyer serves as the Chief for Burn Medical Countermeasures, focused on development of medical countermeasures (MCMs) for burn injuries at the Chemical, Biological, Radiological, and Nuclear (CBRN) threat program within the Biomedical Advanced Research and Development Authority (BARDA), part of the Office of the Assistant Secretary for Preparedness and Response (ASPR) within the U.S. Department of Health and Human Services. Iyer has professional experience in both the biotechnology industry and the U.S. government at BARDA, where he has worked since 2008. Within CBRN, he is responsible for providing strategic direction to the Burn Program toward development and eventual deployment of critically needed MCMs for burns and blast injuries. His program specifically focuses on aligning development of new products toward market sustainability and adopting new products into routine clinical care to generate immediate impact. Products under development in the Burn Program specifically address the challenges in current routine burn- and blast-injury care and increase in overall long-term national preparedness for mitigating consequences from mass casualty incidents with large cases of burn and blast injuries. His experience also covers MCM development for cutaneous radiation injuries and gastrointestinal radiation injuries. He has also served as the acting chief for the Anthrax Vaccines branch of CBRN.

Iyer provides technical guidance for a team that manages projects receiving funding for advanced research and development under Project BioShield, including establishing strategies for procurement and market adoption of MCMs. He works closely with other ASPR offices, the Strategic National Stockpile, the CDC, and review divisions within the FDA that are focused on MCMs to support integration and decisions related to burn and trauma MCM products for use and deployment. He is part of many interagency teams and working groups within the Public Health Emergency Medical Countermeasures Enterprise and DoD that are dedicated to the advancement of MCMs for burns, trauma, and other consequences of a mass casualty. He works closely with the end-user community of surgeons from the ABA and the ACS Committee on Trauma to ensure that the products under development have a meaningful impact. In addition, working with health economists, he has developed working models for evaluating the cost-effectiveness analysis modeling of products under development to provide an assessment of the impact and value propositions of BARDA's investments in burn care.

Prior to joining the U.S. government, Iyer worked as a senior development scientist at Corning, Inc. and in technical operations in the biotech industry. He also worked at Intercell USA, where he was responsible for both early and advanced product development. Iyer received his doctoral degree in molecular microbiology, working as a United Nations Educational, Scientific and Cultural Organization fellow at Biological Research Center in Szeged, Hungary, from the Indian Institute of Science in Bangalore, India. He has many publications from his research at the University of Texas Southwestern Medical Center in Dallas, Texas, and the Johns Hopkins School of Medicine in Baltimore, Maryland.

Amanda Reichard, Ph.D.

Dr. Amanda Reichard serves as a project officer at NIDILRR, a federal organization that provides competitive grants to researchers who share their mission, including those interested in improving the lives of burn survivors. One of Reichard's largest roles is as the program manager for NIDILRR's Burn Model System Program, an interdisciplinary rehabilitation and research program to improve care and long-term outcomes for individuals with burn injuries. She regularly interacts with federal, state, university, and community partners to help improve community living for people with disabilities of all types. Additionally, she conducts health services research regarding health care access and health disparities of people with disabilities.

Planning Committee

This meeting was made possible because of the guidance, planning, and insights of the members of the planning committee of the ninth SoSM:

Dr. Heather Agler
U.S. Food and Drug Administration

Edward Brown
U.S. Army Medical Materiel Development Activity

Dr. Jill Cancio
Center for the Intrepid

Dr. Leopoldo (Lee) Cancio
U.S. Army Institute of Surgical Research

COL Michael Davis
Combat Casualty Care Research Program

Dr. Christopher Dearth
Extremity Trauma and Amputation Center of Excellence

Janelle Hurwitz
BARDA

Dr. Narayan Iyer
BARDA

Dr. Dayadevi Jirage
Military Infectious Diseases Research Program

Dr. Jill Lindstrom
U.S. Food and Drug Administration

Kristin Jones Maia
U.S. Army Medical Materiel Development Activity

Dr. Bonnie Woffenden
U.S. Army Medical Research and Development Command

References

Asif, Bilal, Abdul Rahim, Justine Fenner, Fubao Lin, Douglas Hirth, John Hassani, Steven A. McClain, Adam J. Singer, Marcia G. Tonnesen, and Richard A. F. Clark, "Blood Vessel Occlusion in Peri-Burn Tissue Is Secondary to Erythrocyte Aggregation and Mitigated by a Fibronectin-Derived Peptide That Limits Burn Injury Progression," *Wound Repair and Regeneration*, Vol. 24, No. 2, May–June 2016, pp. 501–513.

Barillo, David J., Morano Pozza, and Mary Margaret-Brandt, "A Literature Review of the Military Uses of Silver-Nylon Dressings with Emphasis on Wartime Operations," *Burns*, Vol. 40, Supp. 1, December 2014, pp. S24–S29.

Cancio, Leopoldo C., Robert L. Sheridan, Rob Dent, Sarah Gene Hjalmarson, Emmie Gardner, Annette F. Matherly, Vikhyat S. Bebarta, and Tina Palmieri, "Guidelines for Burn Care Under Austere Conditions: Special Etiologies: Blast, Radiation, and Chemical Injuries," *Journal of Burn Care & Research*, Vol. 38, No. 1, January–February 2017, pp. e482–e496.

Despa, F., D. P. Orgill, J. Neuwalder, and R. C. Lee, "The Relative Thermal Stability of Tissue Macromolecules and Cellular Structure in Burn Injury," *Burns*, Vol. 31, No. 5, August 2005, pp. 568–577.

Engel, Charles C., Ryan K. McBain, Samantha McBirney, Sara E. Heins, Molly M. Simmons, Emily Hoch, Mimi Shen, Nicholas Broten, Gulrez Shah Azhar, and Tepring Piquado, *The Effect of Blast-Related Burn Injuries from Prolonged Field Care to Rehabilitation and Resilience: A Review of the Scientific Literature*, Santa Monica, Calif.: RAND Corporation, RR-A807-1, 2020. As of October 8, 2020:
https://www.rand.org/pubs/research_reports/RRA807-1.html

Frame, Mary D., Fubao Lin, Anthony M. Dewar, and Richard A. F. Clark, "Vasoactive Effect of Fibronectin-Derived Epiviosamine-1 and Related Peptides in Quiescent and Stress Models," *Microcirculation*, Vol. 24, No. 6, August 2017.

Gomez, Ruben, Clinton K. Murray, Duane R. Hospenthal, Leopoldo C. Cancio, Evan M. Renz, John B. Holcomb, Steven E. Wolf, and Charles E. Wade, "Causes of Mortality by Autopsy Findings of Combat Casualties and Civilian Patients Admitted to a Burn Unit," *Journal of the American College of Surgeons*, Vol. 208, No. 3, March 2009, pp. 348–354.

Greer, Nancy, Nina Sayer, Mark Kramer, Eva Koeller, and Tina Velasquez, *Prevalence and Epidemiology of Combat Blast Injuries from the Military Cohort 2001–2014*, Washington, D.C.: U.S. Department of Veterans Affairs, February 2016. As of October 8, 2020:
https://www.ncbi.nlm.nih.gov/books/NBK447477/

Iyoho, Anthony, Laurel Ng, and Philemon Chan, "The Development of a Probabilistic Dose–Response for a Burn Injury Model," *Military Medicine*, Vol. 182, Supp. 1, March 2017, pp. 202–209.

Johnson, Benjamin W., Andrew Q. Madson, Sarah Bong-Thakur, David Tucker, Robert G. Hale, and Rodney K. Chan, "Combat-Related Facial Burns: Analysis of Strategic Pitfalls," *Journal of Oral and Maxillofacial Surgery*, Vol. 73, No. 1, January 2015, pp. 106–111.

Knox, Francis S., III, *Predictability of Burn Depth: Data Analysis and Mathematical Modeling Based on USAARL's Experimental Porcine Burn Data*, Shreveport, La.: Louisiana State University School of Medicine, 1979. As of October 23, 2020:
https://apps.dtic.mil/sti/citations/ADA091676

Knox, F. S., III, Dena Bonetti, and Chris Perry, *User's Manual for BRNSIM/BURNSIM: A Burn Hazard Assessment Model*, Fort Rucker, Ala.: U.S. Army Aeromedical Research Laboratory, USAARL Report No. 93-13, 1993. As of October 23, 2020:
https://apps.dtic.mil/dtic/tr/fulltext/u2/a438571.pdf

Lairet, Julio R., Vikhyat S. Bebarta, Christopher J. Burns, Kimberly F. Lairet, Todd E. Rasmussen, Evan M. Renz, Booker T. King, William Fernandez, Robert Gerhardt, Frank Butler, Joseph DuBose, Ramon Cestero, Jose Salinas, Pedro Torres, Joanne Minnick, and Lorne H. Blackbourne, "Prehospital Interventions Performed in a Combat Zone: A Prospective Multicenter Study of 1,003 Combat Wounded," *Journal of Trauma and Acute Care Surgery*, Vol. 73, No. 2, Supp. 1, August 2012, pp. S38–S42.

Lin, Fubao, Atulya Prasad, Samantha Weber-Fishkin, and Richard A. Clark, "Engineered Fibronectin Peptide Resists Elastase Digestion, Speeds Healing, and Attenuates Scarring in Porcine Burns," *Journal of Investigative Dermatology*, Vol. 140, No. 7, July 2020, pp. 1480–1483.

Lin, Fubao, Jia Zhu, Marcia G. Tonnesen, Breena R. Taira, Steve A. McClain, Adam J. Singer, and Richard A. F. Clark, "Fibronectin Peptides That Bind PDGF-BB Enhance Survival of Cells and Tissue Under Stress," *Journal of Investigative Dermatology*, Vol. 134, No. 4, April 2014, pp. 1119–1127.

Moritz, A. R., and F. C. Henriques, "Studies of Thermal Injury II. The Relative Importance of Time and Surface Temperature in the Causation of Cutaneous Burns," *American Journal of Pathology*, Vol. 23, No. 5, 1947, pp. 695–720.

Murray, Clinton K., "Epidemiology of Infections Associated with Combat-Related Injuries in Iraq and Afghanistan," *Journal of Trauma*, Vol. 64, No. 3, Supp. 1, March 2008, pp. S232–S238.

National Academies of Sciences, Engineering, and Medicine, *A National Trauma Care System: Integrating Military and Civilian Trauma Systems to Achieve Zero Preventable Deaths After Injury*, Washington, D.C.: National Academies Press, 2016. As of October 16, 2020:
https://www.nap.edu/catalog/23511/a-national-trauma-care-system-integrating-military-and-civilian-trauma

Nuutila, Kristo, Lu Yang, Michael Broomhead, Karl Proppe, and Elof Eriksson, "PWD: Treatment Platform for Both Prolonged Field Care and Definitive Treatment of Burn-Injured Warfighters," *Military Medicine*, Vol. 184, No. 5–6, May–June 2019, pp. e373–e380.

Palmiter, David, Mary Alvord, Rosalind Dorlen, Lillian Comas-Diaz, Suniya S. Luthar, Salvatore R. Maddi, H. Katherine O'Neill, Karen W. Saakvitne, and Richard Glenn Tedeschi, "Building Your Resilience," American Psychological Association, 2012. As of October 16, 2020:
https://www.apa.org/topics/resilience

Parry, Ingrid, and Scott Dewey, *A Goniometry Paradigm Shift to Measure Burn Scar Contracture in Burn Patients*, Tacoma, Wash.: Geneva Foundation, 2019. As of October 21, 2020:
https://apps.dtic.mil/sti/citations/AD1093984

Popivanov, Georgi, V. M. Mutafchiyski, E. I. Belokonski, A. B. Parashkevov, and G. L. Koutin, "A Modern Combat Trauma," *Journal of the Royal Army Medical Corps*, Vol. 160, No. 1, March 2014, pp. 52–55.

Singh, Ajay K., Noah G. Ditkofsky, John D. York, Hani H. Abujudeh, Laura A. Avery, John F. Brunner, Aaron D. Sodickson, and Michael H. Lev, "Blast Injuries: From Improvised Explosive Device Blasts to the Boston Marathon Bombing," *RadioGraphics*, Vol. 36, No. 1, 2016, pp. 295–307.

Tompkins, Ronald G., "Survival from Burns in the New Millennium: 70 Years' Experience from a Single Institution," *Annals of Surgery*, Vol. 261, No. 2, February 2015, pp. 263–268.

Wolf, Stephen E., "Comparison Between Civilian Burns and Combat Burns from Operation Iraqi Freedom and Operation Enduring Freedom," *Annals of Surgery*, Vol. 243, No. 6, June 2006, pp. 786–795.